AYURVEDA PREGNANCY

USING AYURVEDA FOR OPTIMUM PREGNANCY HEALTH AND POSTPARTUM RECOVERY

JILL C. BLAKE

© Copyright Jill C. Blake 2021 - All rights reserved.

The content contained within this book may not be reproduced, duplicated or transmitted without direct written permission from the author or the publisher.

Under no circumstances will any blame or legal responsibility be held against the publisher, or author, for any damages, reparation, or monetary loss due to the information contained within this book, either directly or indirectly.

Legal Notice:

This book is copyright protected. It is only for personal use. You cannot amend, distribute, sell, use, quote or paraphrase any part, or the content within this book, without the consent of the author or publisher.

Disclaimer Notice:

Please note the information contained within this document is for educational and entertainment purposes only. All effort has been executed to present accurate, up to date, reliable, complete information. No warranties of any kind are declared or implied. Readers acknowledge that the author is not engaged in the rendering of legal, financial, medical, or professional advice. The content within this book has been derived from various sources. Please consult a licensed professional before attempting any techniques outlined in this book.

By reading this document, the reader agrees that under no circumstances is the author responsible for any losses, direct or indirect, that are incurred as a result of the use of the information contained within this document, including, but not limited to, errors, omissions, or inaccuracies.

CONTENTS

Introduction   7

1. What Is Ayurveda?   13
2. Pregnancy Care with Food   44
3. Menstrual Care   57
4. Increasing Fertility   72
5. Finally, You Are Pregnant!   81
6. Monthly Diet Supplements   92
7. Labor and Childbirth   99
8. Postpartum Recovery   107

Conclusion   127
References   133

"The great thing about Ayurveda is that its treatments always yield side benefits, not side effects"

— SHUBHRA KRISHAN (GOODREADS, N.D.)

INTRODUCTION

Ingrid and Karl had been married for 15 years and were trying to get pregnant for 11 of them. Ingrid had one miscarriage, during which she suffered immense pain and discomfort. When she became pregnant again, she was worried about her health and the baby's safety. This was before Ingrid stumbled upon the holistic nature of Ayurveda and its connection with pregnancy.

Ingrid researched and learned that from the perspective of Ayurveda, pregnancy was all about *vata* (a combination of aerial and spatial elements that can cause anxiety and unstable moods) management and living a pure, clean life, enhanced by meditation and spirituality. Nourishment, grounding, stability, and rest are all essential qualities to keep those who qualify in the *vata dosha* rooted. So, Ingrid decided to give herself another opportunity and look into nature and her own soul for answers. She looked at her lifestyle and incorporated

Ayurvedic practices where she could with the help of a qualified practitioner. She followed a simple diet, exercised, meditated, and through her practice and efforts, she had a stable, successful pregnancy.

Ingrid's daughter is 15 years old now. This goes to show that we are miraculous beings, capable of so much, if only we have the right guidance and some faith in ourselves.

THE ISSUES

A mother is a treasure in terms of her capability of continuation of the human race. In Ayurveda literature, *stree* (woman) is regarded as the root cause of progeny. Ayurveda is an ancient science that gives importance to defense of one's health and wellness with the help of curative practices drawn from nature. It looks at the individual as an identity, not a generic part of a mass. In doing so, it engineers curative tactics that are tailored to every individual's specific needs.

As of 2020, The National Center on Birth Defects and Developmental Disabilities reports that birth defects affect one in every three newborns in the United States every year. It also states that birth defects constitute the major cause of infant deaths in the country, accounting for about 20% of deaths each year ("Data & Statistics on Birth Defects," 2020). Inborn defects can be seen as minor, major, physiological, anatomical, or latent problems that may manifest in our children as they grow. Data suggests that 3–5% of all births lead to congenital malformations, 30–50% of post-neonatal deaths occur due to this, 11.1% of pediatric admissions are for infants and children who bear the brunt of genetic disorders, 18.5% are children with other congenital irregularities, and 50% of mental health issues stem from genetic roots (Bagde et al., 2013).

In Ayurvedic philosophy, proper and adequate parental preparation is an essential practice to ensure the health of the progeny. While giving birth is a miracle of life, it is a bodily process that can go wrong, particularly if the health of the mother is compromised. So, I am here to tell you that you truly are not alone. If you are trying to get pregnant without mainstream, invasive guidelines and wish to find fertility solutions in alternative medicine, Ayurveda may be your answer.

You may have tried a host of fertility procedures and had little to no success. You are someone who wants a holistic birth process that extends beyond medical care and shields and protects you, helping you give birth to a healthy, beautiful baby. You may be someone who looks at the body as an entity capable of nurturing and nourishing, with proper care and instruction. You may be someone who desires noninvasive, tailor-made care that will look at you as an individual entity and not a mass product in need of generic care. Finally, you may be interested in the role of Ayurveda in postpartum care.

Let me digress for a minute and introduce myself. I am an Ayurvedic midwife with two decades of knowledge and practice in Ayurvedic philosophy and medicine. I am a married mother of two beautiful, healthy children. In my years of practice, I have delivered innumerable babies using Ayurvedic philosophy and techniques. This has equipped me with a concrete understanding of what works and what doesn't. I've seen mothers go through this transformational process over and over again, and Ayurveda has helped each of them in different ways. The great thing about Ayurvedic practice is that it gives credence to individual identity, so you will not get a mode of care that is made for a million other people. Instead, we look at approaches and alternative practices that are meant for you as a mother.

Throughout this book, you will learn about the science that grounds and roots itself in Ayurveda and how it can change your health for the better and contribute to a sense of wellness. I will talk about ways in which you can apply Ayurvedic concepts so that you have a healthy, fulfilling pregnancy. You will be equipped with solutions to fertility and menstrual issues. You will learn a new way of looking at pregnancy through Ayurvedic literature, which perceives conception and different elements that need to come together as important components contributing to the end goal — which is giving birth to a healthy baby. We will discuss Ayurvedic care during the period of pregnancy, and what lifestyle changes you need to incorporate in order to allow healthy growth and nourishment of your fetus. Finally, we will talk about proper postpartum care with Ayurvedic aids. This will be a journey of self-discovery and finding your inner balance.

My sole aim of writing this book is to enable you to have a healthy pregnancy with the help of Ayurvedic practices. What you will learn has been of help to me countless times in my own maternal crises and in delivering healthy, strong babies. Consider this book as a key to learning about pregnancy in a healthy and holistic manner: something that you will experience at a spiritual, grounding level. This is my passion, and I am so happy to have the chance to share it with you and to hope that my knowledge will guide you through your amazing journey.

1

WHAT IS AYURVEDA?

To many scholars, Ayurvedic principles constitute a repository of knowledge that belongs to the world's oldest healing science. The term has its roots in Sanskrit, an ancient literature form. It literally translates to "the science of life." The origins of Ayurveda date back to 5,000 years ago. It originated in a country called India, to the east of Asia. It is often known as the mother of all healing sciences. It stems from ancient Vedic culture and was taught orally for years by accomplished sages and gurus (masters) to their disciples. As the years passed and humans discovered the art of scripture and writing, Ayurvedic principles came to be imprinted in paper. Much of the natural healing systems that we are familiar with today have their roots in Ayurveda. This includes most forms of alternative medicine like homeopathy and polarity therapy.

Ayurveda is an intrinsically holistic health system which supports you from the time you are born to the end of your physical existence. The Ayurvedic way of life aims to help you derive maximum benefit from your time on this planet by optimizing your health with the aid of interventions that do not just help you physically but also look after your mind, spirit, and inner and outer environments. It places a lot of emphasis on disease prevention and health maintenance, along with a comprehensive, naturalistic approach to treatment.

Ayurvedic literature places a lot of emphasis upon prevention over cure and encourages us to maintain our health by paying close attention to the balance in our lives. It encourages right thinking, a simple diet, developing a mind-body connection, and getting in touch with our unique individual constitution so that we can bring about lifestyle changes that are suited for each of us in our own right. By doing so, Ayurveda encourages each of us to find our individual points of balance.

Think of it like this: No two people have the same sets of fingerprints. In the same way, we also have different patterns of energy. We are made of an amalgamation of mental, emotional, and physical characteristics, each with their own skeletal framework. This framework is determined at our very conception, and it remains the same regardless of our age (Lad, 2016).

When something disturbs this balance, internal or external, it reflects itself as a change in our constitution, which derails us and throws us off our ideal state of existence. This disturbance can be the result of a bad emotional state, poor diet and food choices, weather, physical ailments, stress at work, or a troublesome relationship. Ayurvedic literature asks that we identify the factors which are causing us stress. Once we have understood the triggers, we can act upon them in order to return to our balanced states of being. Essentially, you have to understand and accept that health is order, and disease is imbalance and disorder. Once you have accepted this, you will internalize ways to adhere to a state that favors the former.

SCOPE OF AYURVEDA

Many of us think that the scope of Ayurveda only extends to herbal remedies and hot oil massages, but we must remember that Ayurveda is a science. It has an astonishingly detailed scope which studies the complete health of an individual. This includes everything, starting from internal medicine to pediatrics, geriatrics, rejuvenation, surgery, even sexual health (aphrodisiac therapy, also known as *vrsha chikitsa*). Broadly speaking, Ayurveda has eight major principles which are collectively referred to as *Ashtang Ayurveda* or the Eight Branches of Ayurveda:

- The study of toxicology is known in Ayurvedic literature as *agada tantra.*
- Childhood health and pediatrics is referred to as *bala tantra.*
- General surgery is *shalya tantra.*
- Internal medicine is studied as *kalya chikitsa.*
- Mental health and psychiatry are known as *bhuta vidya.*
- Managing diseases and ailments of the head and the neck are referred to as *shalakya tantra.*
- Fertility treatment is called *vajikarana.*

- And finally, rejuvenation and geriatric care is known as *rasayana*.

For the purposes of this book, we will be delving into fertility health and pregnancy from the perspective of Ayurvedic literature.

THE DIFFERENCE BETWEEN AYURVEDA AND MODERN MEDICINE

Ayurveda and modern medicine differ in terms of their functionality. Modern medicine looks at the symptoms. So, if you have a fever, modern medicine will ask if your chest is congested, if you have a cough, or if your stomach is upset. Ayurveda, on the other hand, will look at your whole body. If you run a fever, it will try to understand how your whole body is feeling.

Modern medicine, otherwise known as Western or Allopathic medicine, has contributed to saving innumerable lives. No one can discount its importance. However, modern medicine understands only one term – disease. Its primary job is to manage the disease and to give you a cure for it. It is generic, in the sense that millions of people with similar symptoms will get the similar medicines. There is no tailor-made method to suit individual requirements. So, if you walk into a doctor's chambers and tell them you feel unwell, they will ask about your symptoms, check your vitals, and write a prescription. The medicines in that prescription will work at only curing your symptoms, regardless of other side-effects on your health.

On the other hand, Ayurveda will look at the root cause of the problem by looking at your whole body instead of just a few symptoms. It will try to understand the nature of the imbalance in your body. This is because Ayurveda believes that there is a root cause to all pain, discomfort, and other ailments (Khatri, 2011).

For example, if you have a migraine, there can be a number of reasons for it. You may be dehydrated. Your stomach may be upset. It may have nothing to do with your physical state of being and be a psychosomatic headache resulting from mental stress and anguish. If you go to a doctor, you get a prescription and a pain killer.

However, an Ayurvedic practitioner will find the root cause of the problem and treat that instead of just treating the symptom. If your migraine is stemming from indigestion, an Ayurvedic physician will treat the indigestion, then proceed to curing the headache. Therefore, Ayurveda looks at eliminating the whole problem, instead of just one aspect of it. It is not a bandage or a temporary fix; rather, it is something that looks to cure every aspect of your being so that you live a healthy and fulfilled life (Khatri, 2011).

THE FIVE ELEMENTS OF AYURVEDA: WHAT YOU NEED TO KNOW

To ease your understanding, let us look at the different elements of Ayurveda as principles of density. Density is the measurement of an object in terms of mass per unit of volume. Of the five elements, Ether is the most abstruse, and Earth is the most conspicuous (Parker, 2021):

- Ether is the state of matter where it seems that all that exists is space.
- If there is some movement in space, it is due to air.
- Transformation happens when matter emits heat and light, which is what fire denotes.
- Water is formed when matter is fluid and liquid — it is something that you can touch but cannot control on your own whims.
- Earth is made up of matter that is solid, tangible, and hard.

Since the five elements are distributed in different proportions, each entity and individual is special (Parker, 2021).

The concept of ether is much like that of empty space. Think of the empty spaces in our homes. Each space signifies something, making the whole an integrated, beautiful thing. It is the void that exists between all things and distinguishes one thing from another, but it also paradoxically connects all things. It is the mental location from which all concepts or possibilities emerge. We can look at ether as the spaces between organs, cells, or any hollow areas in our bodies. We recognize an element based on its characteristics. Ether has bright, spacious, subtle, accessible, smooth, and soft qualities. You would be clear and imaginative if you had more ether in your body and mind.

The first of the five great elements is ether, also known as "*akasha*" in Sanskrit. Since it is the most subtle of the elements, it is placed first. It is the essence of emptiness and is commonly referred to as "space." It is the empty space that the other elements occupy. *Shabda* is the source of ether. *Shabda* is the *tanmatra* of sound, which means it is sound in its most basic, unmanifested form. *Shabda* is the primordial space where sensation arises long before it manifests as sound in the ear. The two elements of sound and ether are inextricably linked (Parker, 2021).

The ear is the associated sense organ of the element ether, and the voice (mouth) is its organ of operation, due to their close association. Hearing loss and a loss of voice are common problems caused by an abrogated ether factor in the body (Halpern, 2010).

Ether is responsible for allowing change and growth to occur during the embryo's development. Ether makes space for the other components to come in. The corruption of ether in the body causes a decrease in structure and an increase in space. Tissue is destroyed because of this process. Parkinson's disease is an example of a disorder in which cellular structure is lost and space is generated in the body. The substantia nigra of the brain stem loses dopamine-producing cells, resulting in a rise in emptiness. The loss of islet cells causes a similar situation in the pancreas.

The concept of motion is represented by air. It symbolizes all of the world's energies that have the power to move things. The air theory governs gravity, thermodynamics, propulsion, celestial powers of the moon, and tides. We can't see air in the body, but we can see the impact. The air theory governs nerve impulses, circulation, joint movement, nutrient transport into and out of cells, and waste removal. Air has the characteristics of being cold, dry, rough, erratic, and transparent.

As the inherent potential within space is activated, the element of air is generated. The potential for motion, or kinetic energy, is represented by the element air. *Sparsha* is the source of air. The *tanmatra* – primordial, unmanifested form – of touch is *Sparsha*. *Sparsha* is the most subtle expression of the touch experience's potential. Touch and air are inextricably linked (Halpern, 2010). The skin (through which we obtain touch) is called the element air's associated sense organ due to their close connection. Its related action organs are our hands (through which we reach out and touch the world).

Air manifests itself in the body as motion and life. It is the force that allows blood to pump, nerve impulses to glide, thoughts to circulate, breaths to course, and joints to propel us through life. All motion is propelled by air. Aberrant motion is caused by disturbances in the functions of air. Air may move too quickly, too slowly, or become obstructed. Depending on the position of the disturbed air, each incident has a different effect.

When we think of fire, our minds conjure up images of flame, light, and transformation. Fire is the force that changes something into something else. It is needed in the body to digest and break down food. The principles behind fire are responsible for the transformation of food into body tissue. In the mind, fire also induces wisdom and comprehension. When we say somebody is "luminescent" we are referring to their ability to see things clearly. This trait is made possible with a balanced presence of fire in the body.

The concept of fluidity and flow is represented by water. Plasma, urine, saliva, fluid secretions, and the fluid surrounding cells make up the fluid in the body. Deep feelings of connection, affection, empathy, and compassion are all caused by the qualities of water in the mind. If you have a lot of water in your system, you are more likely to get attached to people and things when you are out of control. It has calm, strong, and flowing qualities.

Water is a symbol for fluidic matter and the physics theory of cohesion. Water is the body's shield; it satisfies the body's most fundamental needs. Water shields the ether element from dissolution, the roughness and motion of the air element, and the heat of the fire element. All pain and inflammation in the body are relieved by the water element.

The water element is the antidote to symptoms that could have the opposite features in the body. When you feel too warm, disbalanced, dehydrated, immobile, frustrated, vulnerable, you can sense an obstruction in your way, or your heart feels like it is in pain, you must find it in yourself to seek out the element of water. Many of the negative qualities are caused by a lack of water. Dehydration, dry mucous membranes, dry skin, weight loss, and reproductive tissue weakness result from the *rasa, medas,* and *shukra* being too dry. Urination, sweating, and the development of dry, hard stools all decrease with a dry *rasa*. Furthermore, the lips and eyes become parched.

The definition of "earth" connotes "solidity" or "stability." Bones, muscles, organs, skin, hair, and teeth are all stable structures in the body. Your body would be heavier and denser if you have more soil in your system. When you are in equilibrium, the earth in your head creates steadiness, and when you are out of balance, it creates stubbornness. Cool, dry, strong, stable, sluggish, and rough are characteristics of the earth element (Parker, 2021).

Earth, or *prithvi*, is the most straightforward of the elements to comprehend: it is what you can see, touch, taste, and sound with your five senses. The physical presence of your body, including your bones and teeth, muscle tissue, and fat deposits, is governed by earth. It is what gives you shape and weight, and what keeps you grounded in the tactile world. Earth is the primal, animal, the symphony of life's flow. Check yourself for signs such as a feeling of instability or insecurity, anxiety, or stress. See if you are accumulating excess weight or feeling ungrounded. In these situations, you need a better balance of the earth element in your life (Reist, 2018).

THE 20 QUALITIES OF AYURVEDA

Guna is a Sanskrit word that means "quality." We note various qualities that work together to produce the action of a material in our bodies, the atmosphere, our minds, food and drink, and everything else in life. The 20 *gunas* in Ayurveda are divided into 10 pairs of opposite qualities that are used to classify various substances. In Ayurvedic literature, every experience is the mixture of 20 different qualities or traits, and they add up to everything we see, hear, touch, and experience. An excess or deficiency of any of these qualities can cause health issues and imbalance in our lives. Knowledge of these qualities help in getting an effective diagnosis and treatment in terms of illnesses. Ayurvedic literature believes that if the treatment only looks at the ailment, it is not enough. One has to look at the opposite quality of the ailment – only that can treat and heal it. As we read the traits of each quality, you will see that each has their positives and negatives ("The 20 Gunas," 2020):

The first set of opposing qualities are heavy and light. Heavy is known as *"guru."* It represents sleep, feeling grounded, stability, a center of being, slow digestion, stubborn behavior, and nourishment. Light is known as *"laghu,"* which translates to being alert, attentive, flighty, and anxious. It also manifests in qualities like fear and insecurity. On another plane, it can refer to reduction in bulk.

The second set of qualities are cold and hot. The former translates in qualities like dizziness, disorientation, compression, inertia, anxiety, oversensitivity, phlegm, mucus, slow digestion, lower immunity, chest infection, and inflammation. The latter manifests in qualities such as gastric balance, improvement of circulation, improvement of metabolism, digestion, integration, and cleansing. On the opposite side, it also translates to qualities like ulcers, chronic inflammation, and a quickness to criticize.

The third set of qualities are oily and dry. The former refers to traits like vigor, sympathy, caring, nourishing, manipulation, comfort, smoothness, moisture, and lubrication. The dry subset translates to contractions, cramping, discomfort, dry skin conditions, dread, anxiousness, isolation, seclusion, detachment, repudiation, and freedom.

The fourth set of qualities are dull and sharp. The first comprises components such as painfully slow thinking and actions, bland behavior, relaxed attitudes, cool temperament, silence, peace, fatty and oily foods, and mindful state of being. The latter has components such as spicy edibles, learners' listening, attention, awareness, respect, and understanding, sores, overdoing, concentrating, volume, and sharp intellectual prowess.

The fifth set of qualities are smooth and rough. The former is manifested in components such as fatty cheese, fruits like avocado, oils, lubricants, *ghee*, prevention of osteoporosis and arthritis, and discrimination. The rough quality is manifested in traits like rigidity, carelessness, dryness, ingestion, constipation, and raw vegetables.

The sixth set describes dense and liquid qualities. The former comprises food items like meat and cheese, and traits such as being grounded, compact, stable, and strong. It also means having healthy muscles. Liquid traits cover dilution, water, salivation, coherence, retention of water, and adaptability.

The seventh state is a coexistence of soft and hard qualities. It translates to components such as a delicate constituency, being relaxed and tender, care and love. Hard qualities relate to the presence of tumors in the body. They also denote strength, selfishness, insensitive behavior, callousness, and a rigid outlook to life.

The eighth marriage is between stable and mobile qualities. The former is a static state of being, denoting traits like stability, quietly sitting in one place, strong faith, healing, and obstruction. Mobility denotes subsets like motion, restless attitudes, and an insecure or shaky state of being. It also denotes activities like jogging.

The penultimate pairing is gross and subtle. Gross denotes obstructions and the presence of anything in excess of what is needed. It also refers to obesity and to food items like meat and cheese. Subtle denotes herbs and drugs, medicine like aspirin, and alcohol. It refers to being emotional and looks at a soft state of existence.

Finally, we have cloudy and clear qualities. Cloudy refers to being confused and incoherent, excessive attachment, and a lack of clear vision. Clear refers to being isolated, excessive faith in cleansing, purification, and sanctification ("The 20 Gunas," 2020).

THE AYURVEDIC *DOSHAS*

The three *doshas*, or constitutions, are at the heart of Ayurveda. You can tailor Ayurvedic treatment to your needs once you know the kind best suits you. Most people are a mix of two *doshas*. The *doshas*, according to Ayurveda, are in charge of bodily tissue formation, maintenance, and breakdown, as well as waste elimination and psychological aspects like feelings, communication, understanding, and love. When the *doshas* are balanced, the body's mechanisms are maintained. However, when one of the *doshas* increases as a result of certain dietary and lifestyle behaviors, an imbalance is formed. Ayurveda may aid in the restoration of equilibrium in areas that have been unbalanced.

People are thought to have a mix of *doshas* when they are born. Our physical, mental, and emotional characteristics are typically determined by one or two dominant *doshas*. The dominant *dosha* determines as to why one person might be unable to tolerate heat or fried foods while another has no reaction to them. Each of the *doshas*, according to Ayurveda, thrives on a particular diet, environment, and exercise routine. Modifying diet and lifestyle factors may help to correct *dosha* imbalances. An imbalance can lead to an infection if left unaddressed. An Ayurvedic practitioner can evaluate an individual by taking a personal and family history as well as administering a medical assessment (Dashiell, 2020).

The three *doshas* are *Vata, Pitta* and *Kapha.*

Prone to mood changes, impetuous, and enthusiastic, a thin frame and defining features are the key traits of the *vata dosha*. The large intestine, pelvis, bones, ears, legs, and skin are all associated with this *dosha*. Your ideas switch about from one thing to the next. You have dry, wiry hair and are lean and gangly. You have a lot of mental creativity, but you get bored quickly.

There are some key traits by which you can recognize a predominantly *vata dosha* personality. They will have a thin body frame and find it difficult to gain weight. They may lose weight easily. Their skin is always cold, brittle, and thin. They have fine, frizzy, and dry hair. Their eyes are small with fine lashes, and they generally boast unusual eye color. Their appetites are irregular, and they may often be constipated. They do not sweat too much ("The Ayurvedic Doshas," 2021).

By temperament, people of the *vata dosha* are energetic, indecisive, anxious, and love to create. They can learn and memorize quickly, but they also forget everything quickly. They are talkative and often talk in an incoherent way that is difficult to keep track of. They dislike cold and dry climates. They dislike routines and like it if their life is unpredictable.

People of the *pitta dosha* have a medium build, are well-proportioned, and have a consistent weight. The small intestine, liver, sweat glands, eyes, skin, and blood are all associated with this *dosha*. If you belong to *pitta dosha*, you are likely to have a keen mind and a voracious appetite to match. Your hair is silky, and you have a medium frame. You are enthused and excited about what you are doing. Normally, you enjoy learning (Wong, 2020).

In summary, people of this *dosha* have a medium body frame and developed muscles, and they find it easy to gain and lose weight. Their skin is mostly warm and oily. They are prone to freckles and acne. They have straight, fine hair which runs the risk of premature graying. They have almond shaped eyes that are bright-colored, and a steady, knowledgeable gaze. Their appetite is intense. They can sweat profusely. They enjoy planning and organizing and can be quite competitive. They are articulate speakers and can make clear, sharp decisions. They learn things quickly and do not forget them easily. They are bright, intelligent, driven, and witty. Sometimes, their keenness and smartness can make them arrogant ("The Ayurvedic Doshas," 2021).

The *kapha dosha* is associated with people who are laid-back and easygoing. With a sluggish metabolism, you are more likely to gain weight. It takes time to commit information to memory, but once you do, you won't forget them. Your physical characteristics include a solid, heavy, and strong frame, as well as a tendency to be overweight.

The lungs, chest, and spinal fluid are all correlated with this *dosha* (Wong, 2020).

Generally speaking, people belonging to *kapha dosha* have broad, curvy, and strong builds, and they can gain weight easily. Sometimes, this can become an issue because the weight can be hard to lose. They have cool skin which is oily and smooth. Their hair is oily, wavy, and thick. They have big eyes with thick eyelashes. Their appetite is steady. They sweat moderately and dislike damp and cool climates. They take time to learn but also remember things very well. They have slow, melodious voices and a calm, quiet temperament. If unbalanced, they can become greedy and stubborn. They enjoy routine and leisurely activities (Hope-Murray, 2021).

According to Ayurvedic literature, each of the *doshas* needs a specific diet, lifestyle, and exercise regimen in order to be in balance. The presence of an imbalance is indicative of something being wrong with one of these components. If it is not checked, it can cause illness. In order to find out your *dosha* and to base your life around it, you can consult an Ayurvedic physician.

Now, each of the *doshas* (*vata*, *pitta*, and *kapha*) have five sub-*doshas*. Each one of them has an effect on and regulates our emotional and mental faculties. Additionally, they also influence the function of our organs and other body operations.

Vata and Its Sub-*doshas*

Prana* Sub-*dosha: The life force energy that enters the body through various systems – food, air, spices, beverages, sounds, smells, touch, and all sensory feedback –is defined and governed by the *prana* sub-*dosha*. This sub-*dosha* controls the vitality of every cell in our body as well as every thought we have. Since *prana* is responsible for the preservation and equilibrium of all physiological processes, including the body's overall homeostasis, any imbalance in this sub-*dosha* has the greatest impact on the nervous system. If this sub-*dosha* is out of balance, it is best to use meditation and pranayama activities, as well as herbs which will nurture the nervous system. Prana can also be aligned by getting adequate rest for your body, harvesting blocked emotions, and going for a walk in nature.

Vyana Sub-*dosha*: The heart is the origin of the *vyana* sub-*dosha* . The cardiovascular system, blood, and nutrient distribution are all controlled or "guarded" by this form of *prana*. Cardiovascular complications, body stiffness, cold hands and feet, and a blocked *anahata chakra* (our abilities to love, empathize, and forgive) are all symptoms of a stuck or imbalanced *vyana* sub-*dosha*. Stretching the body, getting massages on a regular basis, and consuming herbs and healthy food items, including oils that are heart supportive, such as hawthorn berry and rose, are all essential ways to get this sub-*dosha* back into health and harmony (Bliss, 2017).

Samana Sub-*dosha*: The *prana* in the stomach and digestive system is governed by the *samana* sub-*dosha*. A balanced *samana* sub-*dosha* determines how well we can assimilate nutrients from our diet and process unused waste products out of the body. This sub-*dosha* may also have a big impact on how we process and "digest" our mental and emotional experiences. In order to balance *samana* in the body, dietary modifications and appropriate exercises may go a long way in helping us.

***Udana* Sub-*dosha*:** The governing prana over the outward expression of energy, feelings, and behavior is *udana* sub-*dosha*. *Udana* is in control of memories, voice, and the inhalation and exhalation of breath. Problems with the lungs, such as asthma, bronchitis, diaphragm upsets like hiccups, frequent burping, or throat conditions like sore throat, hoarseness, and even thyroid conditions may be connected to an imbalanced *udana* sub-*dosha*. When an individual refuses to express themselves, this sub-*dosha* is suppressed, and it can become negatively affected.

Food items and herbs that help to strengthen and soothe the throat, serve as a nasal decongestant, and enhance memory are recommended. This includes horehound, lemon, and cherry bark. This sub-*dosha* benefits from quiet time in nature as well as warm oil treatments on the body such as sesame oil self-massage and *panchakarma*.

***Apna* Sub-*dosha*:** The key *vata* element, *apana* sub-*dosha* , is prone to irregularity. Many of the problems associated with *vata* are caused by an imbalance of this sub-*dosha*, so it is important to be aware of it. It is also referred to as the "descending wind" because it regulates the downward flow of *prana* in the abdomen, which governs such acts as digestion and expulsion, menstruation, reproduction, urination, and ejaculation. Since the incision influences the air pressure and control within this area of the body, navel births and other lower abdominal surgeries may also disturb this sub-*dosha* .

Pitta and Its Sub-*doshas*

***Alochaka* Sub-*dosha*:** The *alochaka* sub-*dosha* controls how we essentially take in light and translate it into different impressions, information, and images. We will achieve mental clarity and deeper spiritual perspectives on how we "see" truth with the help of this sub-*dosha* . When this sub-*dosha* is depleted, eyes become dull, lifeless, dark, and hollow, to the point that you can visualize how someone has lost their desire to live. When this sub-*dosha* is in equilibrium and peace, it is possible to feel clear and assured about one's course and direction (Bliss, 2017).

***Sadhaka* Sub-*dosha*:** The *sadhaka* sub-*dosha* is located in the realm of the heart and the mind, which is where many people believe the soul resides. On a physical level, it has control over the heart's functions, such as pulse and blood flow. On a psychological level, it aids in the processing of feelings and mental ideas, ingesting them for deeper insights into how we live our lives and assisting us in establishing a spiritual direction. This sub-*dosha* is harmed when emotions build up around the heart, blocking the flow of honest speech and preventing one from feeling and living from the heart. When we give too much emphasis to logic and reason, this sub-*dosha* gets affected.

***Ranjaka* Sub-*dosha*:** The *ranjaka* sub-*dosha* determines the physical color of the body as well as the body's excitement and receptivity to being alive. The spleen, liver, and blood are all under *ranjaka*'s control, and diseases that affect these organs are included, such as skin discolorations, cirrhosis, hyperlipidemia, hepatitis, chronic fatigue syndrome, mental stress, and blood problems. If this sub-*dosha* is out of control, the person will be unhappy in life, poor in body and mind, and may even seem disoriented.

Panchaka Sub-*dosha*: The *pitta* of the digestive fires (known as *agni*) is governed by the *panchaka* sub-*dosha* . Its primary function is to break down foods in order to facilitate nutrient absorption. This sub-*dosha* is often considered when converting ideas and principles into functional data and experiences. It is connected to the *bhuta agni*, or the sacred fire of the belly, as well as the *manipura chakra*. When your *manipura chakra* is balanced, your digestive system and metabolism will be in their best functional capacities. Overconsumption of salty, pungent, and sour foods causes it to become unbalanced. It is recommended that you restore balance with the help of herbs like fennel, cardamom, and cinnamon, as well as meditate and drink plenty of water.

Kapha and Its Sub-*doshas*

Tarpaka Sub-*dosha*: The *tarpaka* sub-*dosha* regulates the overall mental qualities of the *kapha dosha*, which includes the brain and cerebrospinal fluid, as well as the lubrication of the brain and cerebrospinal fluid. The *tarpaka* sub-*dosha* helps to instill a sense of equilibrium and steadiness in the body-mind complex by being slow and steady, and grounded in nature; one who is imbalanced in this sub-*dosha* can feel mentally unstable and a hankering for a greater sense of calm or peace in their life. An imbalanced *tarpaka* may also cause dementia and its different phases, as it aids in the storage of all our sensory experiences in the brain. Herbs that help strengthen brain function and plants like aloe which promote overall wellness are good ways to restore balance in this sub-*dosha* (Bliss, 2017).

***Sleshaka* Sub-*dosha*:** The concept and bodily knowledge of stimulation are brought into the joints as synovial fluids by the *sleshaka* sub-*dosha*. This sub-*dosha* can also be thought of as the quality that allows us to move through change in the outside world with ease. Yoga and martial arts, as well as spinning classes and dancing, can help in strengthening the joints and restoring balance in this sub-*dosha*.

***Avalambaka* Sub-*dosha*:** The *avalambaka* sub-*dosha* dictates and regulates the heart and lungs, but it can also be found traveling around the body, assisting in the transmission of essential nutrients to every organ and component. This sub-*dosha* is known as the "King of All *Kaphas*" because of its role in ensuring that the entire empire of the body is nourished and in balance. The entire body, particularly the lungs, will suffer if the body is out of control, so herbs and activities that aid the respiratory and circulatory systems are recommended.

***Kledaka* Sub-*dosha*:** The *kledaka* sub-*dosha* is the last in the list of sub-*doshas*. This *kapha* form can be found in the stomach and digestive system, where it acts as a source of balance and protection and as an acid regulator. *Kledaka* has a clear and safe codependent relationship with *pitta* fires in the stomach, as the two must work closely to allow for the proper breakdown and assimilation of foods and nutrients. Aloe vera is a beneficial herb for this sub-*dosha* because, unlike antacids, it does not interfere with the natural processes of the stomach (Bliss, 2017).

UNDERSTANDING THE CONCEPT OF BALANCE

When your mind and body are in sync, you can choose what will make both feel better, rather than just one of them. Say you have the craving for a bag of chips. Instead of giving in to those cravings, your mind reasons with your body. "I'm feeling pretty bad right now," your mind says, "but the last time I felt like this and ate a whole bag of chips, I felt much worse. This time, what I'm going to do is grab my mat and go to yoga."

You will remember the chips' hard, bloating after-effects on your body, as well as the shame it caused in your mind. This will give you the strength to forego your immediate happiness in order to work up a sweat and experience a better kind of high.

This is not to say that you will never indulge again. It simply means that you will know when your body really wants to indulge, and when you can pass and focus on something else to spend your time. After all, life cannot be a series of indulgences packed one after the other. Balance is key.

You will be able to be your own judge when you have achieved equilibrium. You know the hankering for advice when you don't trust yourself, and how terrible that feels? This will pass. Your body and mind will advise you about how much to eat, work, sleep, socialize, exercise, and rest. If you have been properly handling your body, you will intuitively know what works and what doesn't. When you need soup instead of spaghetti, or some chocolate and a foamy cappuccino, you will know. The more you understand your body's requirements, the better you will be able to nourish it.

Imbalance refers to a situation where one or more of your *doshas* have increased far in excess of what is required to be in a state of equilibrium. While the equilibrium itself consists of a dynamic movement of the three *doshas*, when one goes too high, your system falls out of order. This results in chaos and havoc. The imbalance has a lot to do with your age, the time of the day, your activity levels, your mental state, the season, and the food you eat.

In Ayurveda, your imbalanced *dosha*, or *vikruti* in Sanskrit, is often addressed first. Your predominant *dosha*, also known as your *prakriti*, is the *dosha* that is most likely to get out of control. When seeing an Ayurvedic practitioner to decide your *prakriti* and *vikruti* is the best way to go, there are some classic signs of imbalance in each of the *doshas* that should help you find out where to concentrate your Ayurvedic rituals and diet.

Imbalance in the *Vata Dosha*

The elements ether and air are included in the *vata dosha*. Since it is the driving force behind all things in the universe and in the body, including *pitta* and *kapha*, it is known as the "king" of all the *doshas*. *Vata* is the energy of voluntary and involuntary motion, transmission, and transportation. Since the *vata dosha* controls so much, it is prone to being imbalanced quickly, even in people who do not have a *vata prakriti*. According to Ayurveda, the majority of our health issues arise because of imbalances in the *vata dosha* ("What's My Vikruti? Classic Signs of Imbalance in Each of the *Doshas*," 2018). While you should consult with a professional to know if you have an imbalance in the *vata dosha*, these are some tell-tale symptoms of the same.

- Anxiety, panic attacks, nervousness, and paranoia
- Involuntary twitches, palpitations, tremors, and spasms – you may find yourself stumbling without warning.
- Chronic fatigue where you are always exhausted, and you feel an inherent incapacity when it comes to doing anything. You are slow, demotivated, and sluggish.
- Your nervous system is affected. For example, you are experiencing neuropathic pain.
- Immunosuppression or immunodeficiency in any form
- Your nails are brittle and damaged, and your skin is peeling, dry, and prone to dandruff.

Imbalance in the *Pitta Dosha*

The *pitta dosha*, which includes the elements fire and water, is known as the *dosha* of transformation because it shifts our interactions from one state to the next. The *pitta dosha*, for example, is in charge of our metabolism and the conversion of food into bodily tissues. *Pitta* is also in control of how mental and emotional interactions are digested. Inflammation or acidity in the body or mind are often associated with *pitta* imbalance. Some symptoms that may point out to your *pitta dosha* being out of balance can include:

- Skin rashes, inflamed skin and aphthous ulcers
- Inflammation in different parts of the body – examples include irritable bowel syndrome which can lead to digestive inflammation and arthritis and can cause joint inflammation.
- Severe acne
- Acid reflux, gastric ulcers, and heartburn

- Anxiety and nausea
- An insatiable appetite and the constant desire to eat
- Diarrhea and loose motion
- Excessive body heat
- Frustration, anger, jealousy, irritation, and an overarching need to be perfect
- Redness and soreness of eyes
- Impotency

Imbalance in the *Kapha Dosha*

The *kapha dosha*, which includes the elements of water and earth, is known as the d*osha* of order and connection. While the other *doshas* are more associated with movement, it offers stability, foundation, and stamina. *Kapha* aids in the feeling of peace, satisfaction, and compassion, assists in the tasting of food, creates and sustains all bodily tissues, stimulates our joints and mucous linings, and protects all our bodily systems and their functioning ("What's My Vikruti? Classic Signs of Imbalance in Each of the *Doshas*," 2018). Stagnation and heaviness in the mind or body are common symptoms of *kapha* imbalances. If your *kapha* is imbalanced, you may experience:

- Excessive mucus in the lungs
- A thick, white coating forming at the base of your tongue
- Infrequent bowel movements
- A desire to eat whenever you are depressed or sad
- A high body weight, with the propensity to gain weight quickly

- Trouble waking up in the mornings, and a desire to sleep all the time
- Feelings of sluggishness, fogginess, dullness, and heaviness
- Feelings of jealousy and being overly attached to people and possessions
- Excessive stubbornness and complacency
- Ovarian cysts, endometriosis, and an enlarged prostate

While you should take the help and advice of an Ayurvedic practitioner to find and tackle the imbalance in your *doshas*, there are some remedies for each of these imbalances ("What's My Vikruti? Classic Signs of Imbalance in Each of the *Doshas*," 2018).

If your *vata* is imbalanced, you should center your meals and routines around foods and practices that are grounding, warming, lubricating, moisturizing, and relaxing. Excess *vata* is balanced by sweet, sour, and salty tastes.

Cooling, relaxing, relinquishing, and restraint are all important aspects of *pitta* pacification practices. Excess *pitta* is balanced by sweet, bitter, and astringent tastes.

Arousal, activity, softening, warming, and drying are all part of a *kapha* appeasing regimen. Pungent, bitter, and acerbic flavors can help to balance a high *kapha* constitution.

THE SEVEN *DHATUS*

According to *Sankhya* philosophy, the world is made up of only two supreme entities: the *purusa*, or spirit, and the *prakriti*, or primordial/primaeval matter (something that has been in existence from the beginning of time). Though primeval matter manifests as five elements that make up the unveiled aspects of the physical universe, it is these five elements that go on to form the three *doshas* that drive all of our body and mind processes and decide our physiological and behavioral makeup right from conception.

Dhatus are the constituent elements that give the body its structure and protection. *Rasa* (plasma), *rakta* (blood), *mamsa* (muscle tissues), *medas* (fat tissues), *asthi* (bone tissues), *majja* (bone marrow), and *shukra* (reproductive organs) are seven types of tissue systems in our body (Chowdhury, 2021). Starting with the *rasa dhatu*, nutrients from food, known as *ahara rasa*, are passed into each stage of the *dhatus* for our body's nourishment. The *doshas* which we derive from what we eat enter the tissue systems (*dhatus*), and the *dhatus* gather the corrupted *doshas* before the imbalance becomes too much and manifests as diseases (Chowdhury, 2021).

Rasa Dhatu

Rasa is the nature of the food that has been digested and absorbed by the body; *rasa* is the food that we are given. It is the first *dhatu* and is derived directly from food, and it serves as the foundation for all other *dhatus*. When consumed in the recommended amounts, it can make one feel satiated on both physical and psychological levels.

The body's fluids, such as menstrual fluid or nourishing breast milk, may be connected to *rasa dhatu*. The intensity of our digestive metabolism, or *jatharagni*, and the quality of the food we consume determine the quality of *rasa dhatu*.

Poor metabolism can degrade *rasa dhatu* quality and make a person drowsy; it has the potential to cause nutritional deficiencies and *kapha* related ailments. The *rasa dhatu* is also depleted by an excess of *vata* and *pitta dosha*, which causes it to dry out. Skin that is dry and cracking, as well as chapped lips, indicate a lack of *rasa dhatu* in the body.

Rakta Dhatu

Simply put, *rakta* refers to the color of blood. The *rakta dhatu* is responsible for the body's tone, appearance, and power. The fire that provides energy and vitality to the body organs and the mind is carried by *rakta dhatu*. It is primarily composed of the element of fire and is aided by *pitta dosha*. *Rakta dhatu* deficiency causes a decrease in body heat and decreased *pitta*, which impairs mental functions such as cognition and memory (Chowdhury, 2021). Excessive amounts of this *dhatu* can cause skin problems and autoimmune diseases including rheumatoid arthritis.

Mamsa Dhatu

Mamsa is a Sanskrit word that means "flesh." *Mamsa dhatu* is responsible for the formation of our muscles, skin, and ligaments. It bears qualities like heat, strength, dryness, stiffness, and heavy density because it is made up of earth and fire elements. When in equilibrium, the *pitta* and *kapha doshas* provide structure, harmony, and homogeneity to the *mamsa dhatu*. Excess and imbalanced *mamsa dhatu* can cause tumors, carcinomas, and cysts, while a lack of *mamsa dhatu* can result in fatigue and weakness. To have solid muscles and healthy skin, you must consume foods rich in earth elements and maintain a healthy metabolism.

Medas Dhatu

The fat that gives luster to the skin, provides moisture and hydration to various parts of the body – including bones and joints – and stores energy to sustain the body is known as *medas dhatu*. Water is the most important component of the *medas dhatu*, as it is the source of nourishment for fatty tissues.

Excessive *medas dhatu* causes fat deposits in the abdomen and other parts of the body. A poor quality or quantity of *medas dhatu* not only leads to obesity, fatty liver, and heart problems, but it also makes the body and mind heavy and sluggish. *Medas dhatu* deficiency, on the other hand, causes the body to become overly thin and the skin and hair to become dry (Chowdhury, 2021).

Asthi Dhatu

Bones are referred to as *asthi* in Sanskrit. The skeletal system, or *asthi dhatu*, is what gives the body its foundation or solid structure. *Asthi dhatu* also forms the teeth in addition to the bones. Excessive *asthi dhatu* formation can cause bone hypertrophy and hyper calcinosis, while a lack of it can cause osteoporosis, joint problems, hair loss, fatigue, brittle hair, bad teeth, and fragile bones. An individual with a healthy and balanced *asthi dhatu* is decisive and optimistic, whereas someone with an unhealthy proportion of the same is stubborn, indecisive, and insecure.

Majja Dhatu

The literal translation of *majja* is "bone marrow." The tissue that carries electrical impulses in the nervous system is made up of *majja dhatu*. It fills in the gaps in the bones, the brain cavity, the spine, and the nerve channels. *Majja dhatu* is also used to make the sclera of the eye and sclerotic fluids. The metabolic process of *majja dhatu* formation also produces waste products in the form of eye secretions. A healthy *majja dhatu* gives an individual a sense of completeness and helps them to be more centered and compassionate.

Shukra Dhatu

Shukra dhatu is associated with male reproductive tissues such as sperm and semen, and female reproductive tissues such as the ovum. The *shukra dhatu* is the most refined of the dhatus. It incorporates the essence of all the other *dhatus*. *Shukra dhatu*, when in balance, encourages creativity and the desire to complete or reach an aim or a goal, but when it is in excess, it can stifle one's innovative spirits (Chowdhury, 2021).

When it comes to our lives, each of us have the unique ability to intake tangible and intangible energies through our sensory organs. When these energies are made for each other, they support the basis of survival. However, if they go against the grain of our individual needs, they result in suffering, disharmony, and disease.

Ayurvedic literature proposes that we correct an imbalance in the body by introducing something that opposes the quality of the imbalance. Consider this simple example: You have the habit of watching thriller movies before sleeping. This gives you nightmares when you fall asleep and becomes a form of suffering. Instead, you switch to watching something calming, reading a book of poems, or doing nothing at all and go to bed with the sole intent of a good night's rest. This results in sweet, dreamless sleep.

Ayurveda offers tailored feedback on routine and seasonal habits, such as the best times to wake up and sleep, as well as how and what to eat for proper digestion and expulsion. Ayurveda uses an extensive repository of herbs when medicines are required. These medications are usually gentler than prescription drugs, and they perform better when used in conjunction with a comprehensive diet and lifestyle plan.

Now that we have established a comprehensive understanding of the foundations of Ayurvedic literature, let us move on and discuss how it may help you in one of the most wonderful phases of your life.

2

PREGNANCY CARE WITH FOOD

In the West, we have devised a variety of methods for determining the nutritional value of the foods we consume. Our diet is often based on a percentage of a prescribed daily allowance, from calorie, fat, and carbohydrate counting to enumerating minerals and trace nutrients. This can all be very confusing and obsession-inducing, particularly if you are trying to balance your *doshas* with a healthy diet!

In Ayurveda, the focus is on the consistency of food taste and how those tastes communicate with the individual's physiology. Ayurvedic literature delineates six major tastes. The flavor profiles are salty, sour, astringent, bitter, sweet, and pungent ("6 Different Types of Taste & Their Roles According to Ayurveda," 2021).

The sweet taste, which combines the elements of earth and water, blends *vata* and *pitta dosha* in the body while increasing *kapha dosha*. This is said to be the most nourishing of the six forms of tastes. They are known to provide durability, resilience, and safe body fluids when consumed in moderation. Be careful not to overdo it, as it can lead to weight gain, obesity, and type 2 diabetes, among other health issues. A majority of our lifestyle diseases are the result of imbalance in terms of consuming this flavor profile.

The sour taste is known to stimulate *pitta* and *kapha doshas* in the body while decreasing *vata dosha*. It is made up of the energies of water and fire. Fruits and vegetables with a sour taste have been shown to improve appetite and saliva production. The sour taste is one of the six distinct forms of tastes that exists, and it is known to awaken thoughts and emotions while also encouraging digestion. It should be consumed in moderation. Lemon, vinegar, pickled vegetables, and tamarind, among other foods, have a sour taste.

Earth and fire forms the foundation of food items that are intrinsically salty. This taste causes *vata* to decrease while *pitta* and *kapha doshas* increase. Salty taste, one of the six tastes in Ayurveda, helps digestion and tissue cleansing due to its hydrating aspect. However, too much of it will raise blood pressure and have an adverse effect on your skin and tissues. As a result, it is best to consume it in moderation. Sea vegetables, sea salt, and black olives are a few examples of salty food items.

The pungent taste is made up of the elements fire and air, and it is the spiciest of the six tastes in Ayurveda. It is used to help digestion, increase appetite, detox tissues, and boost the immune system.

Pungent taste also helps to balance *kapha*, but if consumed in larger quantities than recommended, it can aggravate *pitta* and cause other health problems. When sweet, sour, or salty foods are mixed with *vata*, the result is a pungent taste. Chili, garlic, ginger, sweet peppers, and onions are some food items that belong to this family.

The bitter taste, which is made up of the elements of air and space, is the coolest of the six tastes. It is naturally detoxifying and purifying, and it aids in the removal of toxic waste material from the body. Bitter tastes are best for *pitta* and *kapha doshas*. Turmeric, green vegetables, and herbal teas are examples of bitter-tasting foods.

Finally, astringent taste is defined as cold, firm, and dry and is made up of air and earth elements. People with *vata dosha* should consume this flavor profile in moderation because it can cause flatulence in them. It is beneficial to people who belong to the *pitta dosha*. Astringent food items include unripe bananas, cranberries, and green beans, among others. Unripe bananas can be made into a curry with the balance of other flavor profiles ("6 Different Types of Taste & Their Roles According to Ayurveda," 2021).

LINKING YOUR *DOSHA* WITH THE FOOD YOU EAT

For the *kapha dosha*, pungent food items like onion, ginger, garlic, black pepper, and mustard enhance the appetite, increase digestive powers, and can aid in weight management. Bitter foods such as rhubarb, melon, romaine lettuce, spinach, and chard, as well as turmeric root and fenugreek, are thought to have properties that aid digestion and minimize toxins. Astringent foods such as cranberries, pomegranate, okra, parsley, saffron, and basil can help the body lose excess water, minimize swelling, and promote overall healing. Sweet, sour, and salty foods can be eaten in moderation because too much can cause imbalances in *Kapha*, which we do not want ("*Doshas & The 6 Tastes*," 2018).

Sweet, bitter, and acidic/sharp tastes are the best for balancing and keeping the *pitta dosha* satisfied. Food items with these flavors will help you stay healthy, cool, and calm. Naturally sweet foods include peaches, sweet plums, oranges, melons, carrots, sweet potatoes, and beets, as well as milk and *ghee*, rice and wheat bread, basil, and licorice root. They also have the potential to aid in the growth of healthy tissue. Bitter foods, such as rhubarb, melon, bok choy, romaine and radicchio lettuce, kale, bitter melon, bitter gourd, chard, turmeric root, and fenugreek are thought to have properties that can minimize burning sensations, cleanse the blood, and reduce toxins. Astringent foods such as cranberries, pomegranate, okra, parsley, saffron, and basil can help to reduce fever, avoid diarrhea, and are anti-inflammatory. Salty and sour foods can be eaten in moderation because too much of these can cause a stark imbalance.

Sweet, sour, and salty tastes are the perfect balancing tastes for the *vata dosha*. These flavors will help you stay balanced, grounded, and prevent you from maintaining your body's natural harmony. Sweet food items such as peaches, sweet plums, grapes, melons, carrots, sweet potatoes, and beets; milk, *ghee*, rice, and wheat bread; and basil and licorice root are cooling. They also contain water and earth qualities, which help to ground the airy qualities of *vata*. Sour food items such as yogurt, sour cream, hibiscus, rose hips, green grapes, lemon, caraway, coriander, and cloves are warming, but they also contain the earth factor, which helps to ground *vata*. Salty foods, such as sea salt, rock salt, and sea vegetables are warming and should be consumed in moderation by people of all body types. Where possible, use pink Himalayan salt instead of table salt. Bitter, acerbic, and spicy foods can be eaten in moderation because too much of these food items will disbalance you.

Moderate intake of all six tastes will hold those with *tridosha* (a combination of all three *doshas*) in balance. The key is to limit yourself to just one or two of them. In Ayurveda, the axiom "all things in moderation" forms the crux of all philosophy. Overly sweet, salty, acidic, pungent, bitter, or acerbic foods should be avoided. Remember that too much of a good thing can wreak havoc on your natural body rhythm! Fruits like peaches, grapes, sweet plums, melons, and vegetables like sweet potatoes, carrots, and beets are cooling. Dairy products like milk, *ghee*, and carbohydrates rice and wheat can be consumed in moderation. Seasonings and herbs like basil and licorice root are healthy and possess the potential to aid in the growth of healthy tissue ("Doshas & The 6 Tastes," 2018).

Salty foods such as sea salt, rock salt, and sea vegetables are warming and should be consumed in moderation by people of all body types. Where possible, use pink Himalayan salt instead of table salt. Excess salt can lead to water retention and circulatory problems, causing *vata* and *kapha* to become out of control. Pungent foods like onion, chili peppers, ginger, garlic, cayenne pepper, black pepper, and mustard stimulate appetite, increase digestion, and can aid in weight management.

Bitter foods such as rhubarb, melon, romaine lettuce, spinach, and chard, as well as turmeric root and fenugreek are thought to have properties that can minimize burning sensations, cleanse the blood, and reduce contaminants throughout the body. Astringent foods such as cranberries, pomegranate, okra, parsley, saffron, and basil can help to lower fevers, stop diarrhea, and are anti-inflammatory.

Always check with yourself after a meal. Are you feeling okay? Did you eat just enough? Do you feel bloated or unwell? Are you feeling an acid reflux incoming? If there is any imbalance in your body, it is because of something you ate. So, at every stage, check with your body ("*Doshas* & The 6 Tastes," 2018).

UNDERSTANDING THE SIGNIFICANCE OF THE SIX TASTES

Here is an interesting thing about Ayurvedic philosophy. It links the way we taste food items to the intrinsic nature of the five elements. When you combine ether with air, you have a bitter, astringent flavor profile. If you associate ether with earth, you are left with an acerbic taste, and if you mix it with fire, you get a pungent taste. Similarly, if you combine air with fire, you get an acrid, pungent flavor. If you connect air with earth, the resulting flavor is sour. When you combine water with earth, you can taste a sweet flavor profile. Mix water with fire, and you will taste salty, sour flavors.

I will digress for a minute and look at food from the perspective of modern nutrition. The six tastes satisfy each of the main dietary building blocks from a modern nutritional standpoint. Bitter and astringent foods, for example, are high in vitamins and minerals, while sweet foods are high in fats, proteins, carbohydrates, and water. When our bodies require energy in the form of food, our brain sends signals to our bodies. We will ensure that these signals are properly met by combining all six tastes into each meal. This also aids in the reduction of food cravings and overeating of certain foods ("The Six Tastes of Ayurveda," 2021).

Let's compare two situations from a logical point of view. In the first scenario, you enjoy a balanced meal combining different tastes so that you get ample nutrition from each. In the second, you enjoy a plate of salted fries and ketchup. Your intuition itself will tell you that the latter will result in you feeling hungrier and less fulfilled an hour after you finish eating when compared to the former.

It doesn't have to be difficult to incorporate the six tastes into each meal. A squeeze of lemon, for example, can quickly satisfy the sour taste, while a side salad can quickly satisfy the bitter and astringent tastes. Most of the wisdom of Ayurvedic nutrition is practically on the tip of our tongues, so take advantage of it.

The six tastes assist us in balancing our *doshas* through our diet. The sweet flavor, for example, increases earthy *kapha*, cools hot *pitta*, and reduces airy *vata*. It raises the volume of all tissues because it has a nourishing flavor. As a result, it is no wonder that we eat sweet-tasting foods like oats, root vegetables, and rice to stay healthy ("The Six Tastes of Ayurveda," 2021).

Each taste often influences the body's temperature, either raising or lowering it. Cinnamon, for example, has a pungent and hot flavor that increases body temperature. Grapes are sweet and refreshing, and they can help you cool down. In the same way, something with a hot, spicy flavor profile will naturally contribute to increasing our body's temperature, whereas something that is naturally cooling, like yogurt, will bring it down. When you have a cold, Ayurvedic philosophy will ask that you grind a piece of ginger into your tea – and this will work wonders!

Taste determines whether a food is easy to digest or difficult to digest, as well as whether it is wet or dry on the respiratory tract. Black pepper is a spicy, light, dry, and powerful spice that is easy to absorb, dries mucus membranes, and penetrates deep into tissues.

Here is another unique thing! Tastes have a unique way of aligning with certain parts of the body. We can smell garlic on our (and other people's) breath, so it goes straight to our lungs. Ginger has a variety of effects, including removing mucus from the lungs, warming the skin, energizing the blood, and calming the muscles. According to Ayurveda, asparagus is a bitter, cooling food that helps to clear internal heat through the urinary system. All these examples show that every item we eat is linked with an element of our body ("The Six Tastes of Ayurveda," 2021).

There we have it! The different food items we consume have the ability to reach out and influence the different ways in which our bodies respond to situations. Digestion of food, body temperature, whether we feel good or bloated – every single feeling is connected to what we consume. Our bodies are an intrinsic whole, responding to every item we introduce to them. They deserve our care and nourishment, and that is exactly what we will aim toward.

WHAT'S HOT AND WHAT'S NOT?

Ayurveda classifies foods into three categories based on their nutritional value: *rasa* (flavor), *virya* (power or effectiveness), and *vipaka* (digestive capacity). The coldness and hotness of foods in the Ayurvedic diet are determined by their efficacy. Food items that have a heating effect on our body after consumption are referred to as "hot" foods because they release heat, while food items that have a cooling effect on our body are referred to as "cold" foods because they lower the body's temperature (Jagyasi, 2021).

Ayurvedic care and philosophy is governed by nature's discipline. It provides us with cold foods in the summer to keep our bodies cool and hot foods in the winter to keep our bodies warm. The heating and cooling effects of food are important in preserving good health.

Let's look at some simple examples from food items we consume in our daily lives.

- Vegetables like tomatoes, garlic, ginger, peppers, and condiments like mustard classify as hot food items – cooking oils like *ghee* also fall under this category.
- Fruits like apples, mangos, and oranges are classified as hot food items.
- Cooking spices like asafoetida and *ajwain* are hot food items commonly used to relieve symptoms of fever like cold and cough.
- Fruits like melons, coconut, and vegetables like cauliflower,

asparagus and pumpkin are cold food items that provide strength and nourishment to our bodies.
- Bananas, kiwis, watermelon, apricots, and strawberries are examples of cold foods to enjoy in the summer.
- Most dairy products are also cold food items.
- Hot green tea is ironically a cold food item! It can work wonders for healing and nourishing your body.

When it comes to hot food items, they will aid your digestion and stimulate your appetite. They will also detox and cleanse the body and give you an overall feeling of lightness. However, excessive consumption of hot food items may cause gastritis, chronic inflammation, ulcer, and rashes. On the other hand, cold food items refresh our bodies and cleanse them, all while causing a feeling of drowsiness (Jagyasi, 2021).

The important thing to remember is to eat a variety of hot and cold foods in a healthy manner. We must pay close attention to what we consume and how seasonal variations influence our physical characteristics and eating habits. We gradually develop a compatible relationship with nature as we communicate with food and recognize its constituents and consequences.

HOW DOES THIS CONNECT TO YOUR PREGNANCY?

Pregnancy is a spiritually important period for the mother-to-be in Ayurveda, a time when self-care becomes a concern for both the mother and the baby's health. Ayurveda puts a strong emphasis on maternal care as well as care during and after birth (post-natal care). Due to its holistic nature, Ayurveda considers the physical environment, as well as the mother's mental and emotional well-being, as deciding factors. For a smooth and stable pregnancy, a woman needs emotional stability, pleasure, emotional, physiological, and spiritual nourishment.

Food classification in the modern era is dependent on laboratory results. Even for an informed person, memorizing information about the nutritional value of various foods is a difficult job. Ayurveda takes a simpler route, focusing on three key factors: *tripti* (satisfaction), elimination of hunger, and nutrition.

Ayurvedic philosophy believes that a pregnant woman should consume all tastes, including sweet, sour, salty, bitter, and astringent, while focusing on the Ayurvedic diet based on her individual *dosha* style. The mother's diet must be healthy enough to meet the increased demands, such as preserving her well-being, forming new cells and tissues in the body of the fetus, and supplying the her with the power she requires to give birth and lactate. The mother should be particularly careful with consumption of pungent and spicy food items.

According to Ayurveda, one should always balance their *vata dosha* when pregnant. This is best accomplished by eating a diet rich in organic, plant-based ingredients, whole or sprouted grains, and unprocessed foods. Sweet, freshly cooked foods with healthy oils such as olive oil, *ghee*, and coconut oil should always be consumed during pregnancy. In addition, expectant mothers should stop eating leftovers as much as possible ("Simplify Your Pregnancy with Ayurveda," 2020).

An expecting mother's diet should comprise healthy cereals like quinoa, millet, and whole wheat. You can rely on cooked lentils and pulses. Spinach, kale, amaranth, mint, and fenugreek are good choices of leafy greens. Root vegetables like sweet potatoes, ginger, turmeric, onion, and garlic can be consumed in moderation. Dried fruits like apricots, figs, almonds, and dates can carry you through periods of exhaustion. You can drink green tea or mild white tea with cardamom, cloves, and nutmeg. Fruits like pomegranate, fresh figs, bananas, apples, and avocados are good sources of nourishment. Jaggery can become a good alternative for refined sugar, and rock salt is a good way to substitute table salt. It is better for you to cut back on soft drinks and alcohol completely. Your body must have an adequate amount of vitamin D. This vitamin deficiency causes depression and fatigue, as well as obstructs the immune system. Dairy can be consumed to make up for any deficiency ("Simplify Your Pregnancy with Ayurveda," 2020).

You should always eat what you enjoy when pregnant, but don't forget to eat a well-balanced diet with plenty of fruits, proteins, and healthy starchy carbs. Additionally, keep in mind that you are consuming and nourishing for two people, so you should not follow a single person's diet. As a rule, you should stay away from hot and spicy foods, uncooked leafy vegetables, undercooked beans, and foods containing preservatives and artificial flavors.

If we look at the different food items a mother can consume, we will see that she needs balance most of all. Her diet has to be a balance of all elements and all tastes; if that is achieved, she will have a healthy, fulfilling pregnancy.

In the upcoming chapters, we will go deeper into Ayurvedic care before, during, and after your pregnancy. You will learn the principles of nourishing your body in the way it was intended to be taken care of. In the humdrum and busy flow of modern society, we often forget to return to our roots and look at ourselves as individual beings in need of individual care. Ayurveda is all about reestablishing your balance and harmony with nature, which is how all life is meant to flourish. As we move on, we will seek to provide you with just that.

3

MENSTRUAL CARE

There is no lack of health-related knowledge on topics such as dental care, healthy eating habits, ways to take care of your heart, organs and bones, or how to keep your stomach bacteria functional, but how do you take care of your womb? Why is it even important? Outside of the major transformations of puberty, pregnancy, and menopause, Ayurveda is one of the few disciplines that looks at the reproductive tissues; Ayurveda also examines the menstrual cycle as a window into the human body in a special way. You can understand which *dosha* imbalances your body is dealing with on a month-to-month basis if you are familiar and in touch with your menstrual cycle.

Simply put, the menstrual cycle is a byproduct of the body's most essential tissues. The food we ingest is transformed into usable nutrients so that the body's tissues can absorb and use them for growth and maintenance. Plasma comes first, followed by blood, and then muscle and fat tissues. After these four layers, the reproductive tissues, the nervous system, and the bony tissue follow. Menstrual flow is thought to be a byproduct of the first layer or *rasa dhatu* – also known as plasma. Plasma serves as a delivery system for nutrients. It transports hormones, vitamins, minerals, and water, as well as other nutrients.

Excess *vata*, *pitta*, or *kapha* impairs the quality of the *rasa dhatu* and the *rakta dhatu* after they leave their gastrointestinal tract. You will get a good sense of how the *doshas* are at work even before they completely manifest on a larger level in other layers of the body by paying attention to your flow, its qualities, and your overall experiences (pain, discomfort, or a comfortable cycle) before and after. This allows for intervention such that the body's physiology can be restored to a more balanced state, resulting in better health.

This is one of the most important aspects of pregnancy. The health of your menstrual cycle directly impacts the health of the reproductive system, and an unhealthy cycle can result in a difficult pregnancy or lack thereof.

UNDERSTANDING A HEALTHY MENSTRUAL CYCLE

The expulsion of blood through the vagina of an adult female during a period is known as *artava*. It is one of the most essential physiological processes that allows the *garbha* to develop. In Ayurvedic philosophy, *artava* is the *upadhatu* of the *rasa dhatu*, which means that it is the foundation on which the other *dhatus* build themselves.

Females of today's generation face a slew of issues with their menstruation, including painful periods, erratic cycles, irregular bleeding rates, and more without any apparent irregularities in their reproductive system. For this purpose, Ayurveda philosophizes a healthy menstrual cycle. The menstrual cycle will run smoothly as long as the *doshas* work normally and are not interrupted or overshadowed by another *dosha*.

Ayurvedic literature believes that every individual has their own *prakriti*, which is a constituency determined by the predominant *dosha* in each of them. This influences the occurrence and intensity of different body processes. For instance, pain is a dominating feature in the *vata dosha*, so women falling under this *dosha* are at increased risk of painful menstrual cycles. In the same way, *pitta prakriti* people may be more prone to moodiness, while *kapha prakriti* people may have more clots in their menstrual blood.

Menstruation and your cycle are used as a natural cleansing phase in Ayurveda. Our bleeding days are thought to be a time of rest and rebirth, a time when we can focus more inward and listen to our inner wisdom. Even though our monthly cycle is a perfectly normal phase, many of us regard it as a frustrating and inconvenient experience. Periods are seen as a curse that we women must "deal with."

A healthy menstruation lasts three to five days and occurs every 24 to 32 days, according to Ayurveda. Every woman is different, so if your cycle lasts 26 or 30 days, as long as it is constant and reliable for you, it is considered natural. If your cycle lasts 26 days one month and 32 days the next, you should be on the lookout for any imbalances. Signs of a healthy cycle include

- Bright red color of blood flow
- No stubborn stains in your clothes (stubborn stains can be an indication of toxins present in your body)
- No unpleasant odor
- A balanced flow that is neither too dry and scanty nor too heavy

UNDERSTANDING THE RELATIONSHIP BETWEEN YOUR *DOSHA* AND YOUR MENSTRUAL CYCLE

Ayurvedic philosophy believes that your predominant *dosha* has a lot of influence over your menstrual cycle. At different times during your menstrual cycle, each of the *doshas* plays a significant role. Pre-menstrual, post-menstrual, and menstrual symptoms (ranging from cramps and mood changes to increased appetite and sweating) are all linked to the equilibrium (or imbalance) of the *doshas* in your body. Since the amount of *ama* (or toxins) stored in the tissues influences the intensity of symptoms, one of the most effective ways to restore *sattva* (a Sanskrit word translating to goodness and harmony) to your monthly cycle is to gradually reduce your toxic load. We can do this in a variety of ways, including a balanced diet, gentle exercise, and avoidance of processed or junk food.

Vata Menstruation

Vata personalities are more likely to have irregular, inactive, and painful periods. This is due to *vata*'s constricting, cooling, and tightening effects on the blood vessels. V*ata* also has a natural home in the pelvic space, and if the imbalance isn't corrected, *vata* forms are prone to tissue loss, which can manifest as outer emaciation. Periods can stop for a while for *vata* types who lose weight quickly, particularly if the weight loss is the result of nervousness, breakdowns or emotional turmoil. When blood does appear, it is always darker in color, indicating that older blood from a previous cycle has merged with newer blood and that the flow from the uterus has been hindered.

On every stage, we want to nourish, lubricate, feed, ground, steam, and soften to counterbalance the dry, cold, sparse qualities of *vata*. Return to your childhood comfort foods: sweet, mushy, calming, warming, and fragrant. Soups, stews, and curries (a yielding marigold-yellow *tarka* dal is generally a good option) cooked with plenty of butter, coconut, sesame oil, or *ghee* can nourish those tissues from the inside out. Switch from coffee to calming, warming teas like cardamom and cinnamon, as well as soft, softly spiced milks like golden turmeric milk and chai, which are gifts to the *vata* body.

Pitta Menstruation

Pitta cycles are always heavy, and they can start quickly, with heavy bleeding coming on all of a sudden. This is mostly owing to the heat, flow, and force of *pitta* (which is characterized by the fire and water elements). With the heat comes a noticeable rise in temperature (many *pittas* feel extremely hot and bothered in the days leading up to and during their period), tenderness, and swelling – particularly in the breasts. *Pittas* are more likely to have loose bowel movements and diarrhea during their cycles due to the rush of blood and increased heat in the tissues; many may also feel nauseated and exhausted.

Easing up in all other respects is one of the most effective ways for *pittas* to control their own inner fire during their heavy periods. That means avoiding competitive, offensive, or excessively demanding behavior and activities, as well as any activity that raises your blood pressure. Spicy, excessively rich, oily, and salty foods, on the other hand, can continue to stoke the inner fire when it needs to be quenched and cooled. Mint, nettle, lavender, chamomile, coriander, coconut oil, and coconut milk are cooling food items that you can rely on during this time.

Kapha Menstruation

Kapha is the heaviest and most sluggish of the *doshas*, with earth and water as its components. Their stagnant constituency makes it difficult for items to pass through the body in a healthier way, and *kaphas* are more likely to hold fluid, bloat, swell, and experience bowel and abdominal distention. *Kaphas* have longer periods, and their blood is thicker, stickier, and heavier. An urge to sleep more pervades as well, but unfortunately for *kaphas*, this will only worsen the tiredness.

To restore balance, we pursue lightness and fluidity once more, working with the universal law of opposites. The body needs to be warmed up, excited, and energized if it is excessively moist and cold on the inside, which causes sluggish feelings and slow fluid flow. Now is the time to stoke *agni*, which is the fire that transforms and enlivens us (and drives metabolism). Black pepper, cinnamon, and ginger can all be used to spice up your meals. *Kapha*-elevating food items also include poultry, yogurt, and cheese; light broths, tangy soups, spiced pulse curries, bean curries, and stews; and *tulsi* (holy basil), cardamom, turmeric, and cinnamon Ayurvedic teas are all good choices.

You seem to have painful cramping, bloating, extreme mood swings, or some other kind of pain or discomfort that is far in excess of what is normal – these are all signs of a body imbalance. They may not have anything to do with your cycle necessarily. Your cycles are less likely to be stressful, painful, or have a negative effect on your life if the *doshas* in your body are all in order. This is why Ayurveda focuses on addressing the imbalance at its source rather than only treating the symptoms.

You may not realize this but the imbalance in your body can affect your monthly cycle and disrupt healthy flow. Hormones in your body that regulate your cycle help you get pregnant; maintaining a healthy pregnancy affects things like cycle length, how heavy your flow is, and how regularly you will get your period. When hormone levels are out of whack, which can happen due to underlying medical conditions, stress, or drastic dietary changes, your menstrual cycle is likely to face obstruction. There are several complications that can arise with problematic periods, and all of them have something to do with an imbalance in your *doshas*.

Missing Your Period: There is nothing worse than skipping a period for the wrong reason while you are trying to conceive. If your monthly visitor isn't turning up, well, monthly, and you are not seeing the two pink lines you are looking for, you should see a doctor to figure out what's wrong. This is mainly because an abnormal cycle affects your fertility in two ways. To begin with, pinpointing those crucial ovulation dates when getting pregnant is most likely would be much more difficult. More specifically, missing periods on a regular basis can signify underlying problems that can affect your fertility; some of these issues are significant, while others are easy to resolve. PCOS is the most well-known source of irregular periods. Hypothyroidism, as well as high prolactin levels (increasing breast size and production of breast milk during and after pregnancy), zinc deficiency, excessive dieting or weight loss, or extremely vigorous exercise can all cause amenorrhea.

Abnormal Flow: Menorrhagia (abnormally heavy menstrual cycles), also known as *asrigdara* in Ayurveda, is the underlying symptom that causes a normal menstrual cycle but with unusually heavy bleeding and a longer period, eventually contributing to fatigue and general debility. Most of the underlying causes of very heavy cycles are the same conditions that make it difficult to conceive or maintain a stable pregnancy: uterine fibroids or polyps, endometriosis, pelvic inflammatory disorder, or a hormonal imbalance.

Light Flow: If your light cycle is a sudden shift that isn't explained by increased stress or drastic weight loss, you should investigate what is causing it. Polycystic ovarian syndrome, or PCOS, is a disorder in which women emit more male hormones than normal, and it is one of the main underlying medical problems when it comes to triggering a light phase. Also, as you are probably aware, PCOS can be one of the most common causes of infertility in women today. This may be a sign of a major hormonal imbalance.

Cycle Length: The general interval of menstrual cycles is 28 days. However, since we are all unique, there will always be some difference in cycle duration. It is perfectly normal if one person's period is off by a day or two. Significant variations in cycle duration, on the other hand, may indicate problems such as hormonal imbalance or other underlying medical conditions that can influence fertility. When not on any form of birth control, the length of your cycle can be a key indicator of hormonal imbalances and whether or not ovulation is occurring on a regular basis. Hormonal imbalances can influence when and if you ovulate during your cycle.

Spotting: At some point in their lives, many women will experience unexplained vaginal bleeding or "spotting" in between cycles. This can be brief or seem to go on indefinitely, and it can also stop and start for no apparent reason. Although it does not always mean a significant issue, it may be very inconvenient. Spotting may be caused by a variety of factors, including the use of some medications, such as the birth control pills or other contraceptive devices, or by a reproductive organ infection, PCOS, or STDs. Ayurvedic spotting treatment focuses on hormone imbalance. Ayurveda never tries to artificially add hormones, instead using herbal formulas that enable the body to produce its own hormones. In several cases of vaginal bleeding, signs and symptoms of a mineral deficiency in the reproductive region, such as a calcium or iron deficiency, can be detected, and Ayurvedic formulations can be used to correct the problem. The problem, according to Ayurveda, is caused by an excess of *pitta* in the reproductive system, and the Ayurvedic remedy involves a *pitta* pacifying regimen.

A number of other issues like overly long or short cycles can happen because our bodies are not properly tuned to the harmony and balance of nature. In all these situations, following a holistic diet that draws from all the elements while focusing on your primary *dosha* can give you relief.

A NOTE ON THE USE OF OILS IN AYURVEDIC PRACTICE

The *Charaka Samhita: Sutrasthana*, which is one of the foundational texts of Ayurvedic theory and practice, emphasizes on the holistic nature of massages in restoring harmony to your system. According to the text, massaging oil into the human body gives it sound and vigor in the same way as water gives a tree or plant's roots the nutrients they need and encourages growth. Bathing and massaging your body with oil allows it to enter the system, and sooth and invigorate the body with its essence (Wolf, 2016).

The contemporary urban lifestyle is characterized by physical and mental exhaustion. Such a way of life aggravates the *vata dosha*, which leads to a mind-body imbalance in Ayurveda. *Vata* imbalances cause emotional, nervous, and digestive problems, as well as low energy and body tissue weakness. Taking care of *vata* is important for balancing all of the *doshas*. *Vata* energizes and upholds *dharma* on a cosmic level and balancing your *vata* gives *dharma* or natural order to the body and mind's workings (Wolf, 2016).

Massaging your body with Ayurvedic oils is nourishing for your body for several reasons, some of which are listed below:

- It relieves stress and is calming for the mind.
- It heals and repairs dryness of the skin and the hair.
- It improves your blood circulation.
- It aids in your digestion.
- It eliminates toxins from your body,
- It can give you a lot of relief during your periods, and
- It restores mental cognition and alertness.

Apana vayu is one of the most important concepts related to pregnancy. It is a downward flow of energy in your body that is responsible for menstrual blood flow, toxins, and other expulsions. It has everything to do with the quality and quantity of your menstrual flow. Ayurveda aims to stabilize *apana vayu* so that your cycle is relaxed and does not interfere with your *vata*.

Warm oil baths or *abhyanga*, which involves self-massage, are used to calm the *vata dosha* in Ayurveda. Since sesame is the most penetrating of all the oils, it is an excellent choice for oil baths. Sesame oil drops may be applied to the eyes, nose, and ears. Sesame oil is high in linoleic acid and has antioxidant and anti-inflammatory effects (Wolf, 2016).

When you are menstruating, rub sesame oil into your lower abdomen for relaxation. By binding the *vata dosha* with medicated oil and herbs, you may force it back to its position. This is why daily *Abhyanga* practice during the month has such a significant impact on your menstrual cycles. In simple words, massaging is an excellent way to help you stabilize yourself, both mentally and physically. It can be used at any time to help you center yourself and keep your body in motion. It can help with cramping, water accumulation, exhaustion, and crabbiness that come with menstruation ("Simplify Your Pregnancy with Ayurveda," 2020).

Oil baths include gently massaging each part of the body, including the scalp, with the oil of choice which is pleasantly warm. Allow 10–15 minutes for the oil to soak into the tissues after the massage. The oil massage is usually accompanied by the application of *ubtan*, a paste made primarily of gram/chickpea flour (*besan*), turmeric, and milk. The paste is applied to the entire body (except the head), dried, and then wiped away. After that, the body is just rinsed with warm water and no soap is used.

Dhanwantharam Thailam (oil) is an Ayurvedic medicated oil for *vata* imbalances. It can be used for massage both internally (orally) and externally. Both its internal and external use are helpful in the treatment of paralysis, hemiplegia, quadriplegia, and wasting or physical weakness. It increases the strength of the body's muscles, ligaments, tendons, and other tissues. It is also neuroprotective, so it is essential for neuroprotection and maintaining the nervous system's natural functions. However, in high doses, it may induce side effects such as indigestion and cramps, so always confirm your dosage with a doctor or specialist.

Women should avoid *Abhyanga* during pregnancy. Those who are sick, injured, or have broken or infected skin should also avoid massages unless prescribed. Consult your doctor before taking an oil bath if you have any medical conditions. The *kapha dosha* should also be careful with oil massages because their skin tends to be heavier and oilier than the other *doshas*. If you have a predominance of *kapha* in your body, use lighter oils like olive or almond for massages.

So, with that in mind, what are some things you can do to ensure a healthy period? We will list some tips below ("Ayurvedic Tips For A Healthy Menstrual Cycle," 2018):

- Try to adhere to an Ayurvedic daily routine and a night routine for restful sleep.
- Consume light, easily digestible foods while menstruating.
- Consume foods that are appropriate for the climate and altitude in which you live.
- Eat a balanced diet to maintain a healthy *vata*, *pitta*, and *kapha dosha* balance.
- Use pads rather than tampons.
- Remain as still as possible during menstruation.
- Place the hot water bottle on the lower abdomen to alleviate pain.
- Drink decaffeinated ginger tea if you find yourself bloating.

If you have a strong flow, avoid it and instead make an Ayurvedic detox tea or try *ashwagandha* tea.
- When you are not on your period, do yoga, pranayama, and self-massage.
- Shower instead of bathing during your menstrual cycle.
- Infertility, unusual or painful menstrual cycles, fibroids, ovarian cysts, uterine prolapse, yeast infections, endometriosis, hemorrhoids, constipation, or discomfort throughout intercourse are all treated with vaginal steam baths. It is also used to cleanse and revitalize the uterus, as well as to keep fertility in check. However, only do these in consultation with a medical professional.
- Raw meat, fish, eggs, fast food, caffeinated tea, caffeine, beer, and cold beverages should all be avoided, as should eating before the previous meal has been digested. With that being said, it is best not to miss meals. You can space out what you eat between your main meals, and never overfeed or underfeed yourself.
- To keep the mind quiet, avoid noisy sounds, violent movies, and so on.
- To avoid vitiation of *vata dosha*, avoid fast running and excessive conversation.
- Finally, do not suppress any natural human behaviors like sneezing, urination, coughing, and so forth because suppressing your natural constituency will cause imbalance in the *vata dosha*. *Vata dosha* heads in the opposite direction of its usual downward flow if natural impulses are suppressed.

Remember that your menstrual cycle is part of your body's natural function, and there is nothing bad about it. It exists to protect you. Treat it as you would treat any other function of your body – with acceptance. Don't look at it as something that is there only to give you pain and discomfort because the way we think reflects in some ways on our physical bearings. Focus on correcting your imbalances and leading a healthy life, and this will ease your cycle naturally.

4

INCREASING FERTILITY

Ayurveda offers a comprehensive approach to improving and helping fertility. Fertility in both men and women is being impacted by a variety of factors these days, including stress, pollution, poor diet, and sedentary lifestyles, to name a few. To ensure that the mind and body are in optimal condition to procreate, it is important to cleanse the body of toxins and nourish it with optimal nutrients. After years of trying, one out of every seven couples has trouble conceiving (Karamchedu, 2013). There are many social, behavioral, and physiological causes for this. About 25% of cases may also be unexplained infertility, of which there is no known cause (Karamchedu, 2013).

Fertility and population growth rates are steadily declining around the world, especially in developed countries. The increasing age of women attempting to conceive in busy urban communities, as well as the rising cost of child rearing in nuclear families, is a barrier to fertility rates. Increased use of pesticides and chemicals is also thought to be a contributing factor, particularly in male infertility.

The proportion of couples depending on stressful and expensive assisted fertility methods such as IVF is also growing. In this context, it is important to consult conventional wisdom in Ayurvedic science for guidance in developing a holistic approach to infertility and reproductive health. According to Ayurveda, the most important factors in the pregnancy process are not just healthy sperm and ovum. Greater focus is placed on metabolic function, hormonal balance, and mental/emotional well-being, as well as the relationship between these factors and healthy sperm/ovum.

Fertility increases when the conditions in the world are conducive to the development and growth of a child, and these conditions will vary case by case since each infant, like each parent, has a unique nature, or *prakriti*. There are no two alike. The genome, which is a component of *prakriti*, is a term used in modern medicine. Ayurveda promotes natural peace by linking a person's inner world (mind, body, and spirit) to the outside world (the seasons, environment, and larger macrocosm of all living things).

The ancient wisdom of Ayurveda returns us to the very basic biological concepts that underpin the creation of life. For natural fertility and reproductive health, four fertility factors must be considered: the seed, the season, the fertile field, and the nourishing water.

Beeja **(the seed)**: The reliability and quality of the *beeja*, or sperm and semen, plays an important role in the creation of the *garbha* (pregnancy). Unhealthy diet and activities, stress, and behavioral disorders can all lower sperm quality, resulting in infertility and difficulty conceiving. In today's fast-paced life, living in balance with our inner selves is most important for healthy *beeja*.

Ritu Kala **(the season):** *Ritu kala* is the most fertile time and is regulated by *kapha*. This well-developed proliferative process occurs in conjunction with ovulation. It is the time following menstruation during which the endometrium thickens and develops. When this *kapha*-dominant process is influenced by an imbalanced amount of *vata* or *pitta*, it can interfere with a woman's fertility during the menstruation cycle.

Kshetra **(the fertile land):** The uterus and other reproductive organs that contribute to the development and conception of a fetus and the parenting of an infant, as well as the wider environment surrounding mother, child, and family, are included in the concept of a fertile land. A new baby will make a home in this land.

Ambu **(water):** Water is what flows through the field, nourishing both mother and child's tissues, transmitting messages through hormones, and lubricating the body for the massive physical changes that occur throughout the menstrual cycle, childbirth, and birth. Water acts as an agent of nourishment; it is a carrier and a mixer. It keeps the temperature within the body stable so that metabolic processes may take place within their optimal range.

Conception can become difficult if there is a problem in any of these four fertility areas. The mind, body, and environment are all essential factors to consider when trying to conceive. Your partner's role can never be invalidated, but you are the main act in this show. It is your body that will decide the correct time and environment. Ayurveda focuses on improving a person's daily activities, diet, and lifestyle with self-care and attunement to the environment to affect fertility factors. You plant your seeds, and if everything goes right – at the right time, in the right climate, and with the right care – you will become pregnant. The target here, however, is not simply to become pregnant; you just want the rest of your life and well-being to go as smoothly as possible. One of the most valuable gifts you can offer to someone is your well-being, which includes yourself, your partner, and potentially your future child.

INFERTILITY

In Ayurvedic medicine, infertility refers to a woman's biological failure to contribute to reproduction as well as the condition of a woman who is unable to bring a pregnancy to full term. According to modern science, infertility is described as the inability to conceive after a year of regular intercourse without contraceptives. Infertility is a common issue nowadays, and it has become imperative to find a solution that is both simple and affordable. The ancient literature *Atharvaveda* thoroughly explores the Ayurvedic background on the necessity of treating infertility.

Of course, you may try modern medical approaches to help you if you have trouble conceiving, but you may also find your answers in Ayurvedic thoughts and practices. Infertility may be caused by either male or female causes.

Ovarian abnormalities, tubal factors, age-related factors, uterine disorders, PCOS, endometriosis, and other factors may all be causes behind female infertility. The menstrual cycle can be influenced by a variety of factors, including diet, mental instability, unnecessary physical activity, lifestyle, and stress, all of which contribute to a *dosha* imbalance. At the same time, male infertility is typically triggered by issues that affect either sperm development or sperm transport, such as varicocele, infections, ejaculation issues, tumors, hormone imbalances, defects in sperm transport tubules, and so on.

Ayurveda allows you to heal your imbalances by improving the body's own self-healing and balancing processes, rather than relying on outside or external substances to substitute or correct hormones in the body. It focuses on the systematic treatment of infertility with the goal of improving the individual's overall health and quality of life.

Agni, the principle of fire we explained earlier, is fundamental to Ayurvedic philosophy. In fact, the body's *agni* is one of the most important factors in deciding overall health. *Ama*, on the other hand, is a poisonous, disease-causing agent that develops as a result of damaged *agni*. Unfortunately, *ama* aggregation is particularly harmful to our health; it can cause a variety of imbalances and is a contributing factor in a variety of diseases. Infertility is among these (Mischke, 2020).

Another important Ayurvedic concept is that of *ojas*, or the path to enlightenment. The path to perfect fitness, pleasure, and brain integration is through *ojas*. When you are in good spirits, you can see *ojas* in the shine of your skin or the glow in your eyes. The more *ojas* you have, the more vitality, health, and youth you will have. *Ojas* is also beneficial to boosting immunity and building resistance to disease ("Ojas," 2015).

Infertility does not exist in isolation. It is, rather, a culmination of illnesses. As a result, the herbs used in the procedure are aimed at eliminating the root cause. The most well-known and widely used herbs, such as *ashwagandha (Withania somnifera)*, *shatavari (Asparagus racemosus)*, and *amalaki (Emblica officinalis)*, are extremely beneficial Ayurvedic herbs that aid in the development of a symbiotic hormonal equilibrium. No single herb is thought to be useful for encouraging fertility. As a result, in the treatment of infertility, a mixture of herbs is used with the aim of correcting an organic or functional condition that induces infertility ("Infertility Management in Ayurveda," 2019).

Ayurvedic herbs used in infertility treatment differ in terms of the different conditions involved. For example, problems related to ovulation are treated with *ashoka, dashmoola, shatavari*, aloe vera, *guggulu*, among other herbs. Premature ovarian failure (POF) can be cured with *ashoka, dashmoola, shatavari, guduchi*, and *jeevanti*. Fallopian tube blockage, adhesions and lesions (scar tissue), and pelvic inflammatory disorder can be healed with *guduchi* and *punarnava* ("Infertility Management in Ayurveda," 2019).

The right mix of herbs aids in managing menstrual cycles, optimizing general health and well-being, revitalizing sperm (improving a man's sperm count, morphology, and motility), mitigating stress, improving sleep, controlling anxiety, increasing energy levels, balancing the endocrine system, and improving blood flow in the pelvic cavity, all of which contribute to fertility.

Another way to uplift your mind and body can be through massages. Massaging revitalizes the entire body, decreases fatigue, and balances the underlying *dosha*. Female infertility may be affected by pelvic adhesions, blocked channels, or other forms of damage or inflammation in the reproductive system. Although conventional medical knowledge has always considered surgery as the only way to alleviate these issues, massage therapists have discovered that deep tissue massages can not only remove mechanical obstructions but also reduce pelvic pain and increase sexual desire and orgasm in women (Karamchedu, 2013).

Another aid is through the practice of fertility yoga. Fertility yoga is a form of yoga that is intended to help couples who are having trouble conceiving. It adheres to the fundamental concepts of yoga, but also mixes conventional yoga postures with postures that have been deliberately designed to enhance an individual's reproductive health, thus improving their odds of becoming pregnant.

Yoga for pregnancy increases both female and male infertility by reducing tension, which balances the body's hormones as well as one's mental well-being, improving the potential to conceive for a couple.

In addition to the stress-relieving effects that aid pregnancy, fertility yoga benefits optimal health and wellness in the following ways (Karamchedu, 2013):

- The body is strengthened and toned.
- Increases the supply of blood to the uterus and ovaries
- Reduces inflammation in the body
- Aids in improved breathing
- Increases adaptability to the changing environment around us
- Balances appetite, boosts libido, alleviates depression, and makes you feel more in control of your body

Ayurvedic practice requires you to bring balance to your body even before you are in the stage of conception. This begins with *ahara rasayana,* or a thorough evaluation of the mother's digestive system, and the suggestion of appropriate measures to enhance digestive function. At least three months prior to conception, the parents must practice routine cleansing of their bodies in order to wash off environmental pollutants and toxins. This function, also known as *vihara rasayana,* can be practiced with gentle yoga, breathing exercises, walks in nature, and meditation. *Achara rasayana,* or the reading of good books and engaging in uplifting conversation, is to be done by the mother-to-be. Finally, *aushadha rasayana,* or Ayurvedic herbal remedies, can provide balance to the mother before her conception. In all these situations, the parents must take the prior advice of a professional (Douillard, 2020).

Finally, we have *panchakarma*, which corrects imbalances by removing harmful *amas* from the system. *Panchakarma* therapy consists mostly of regular massages and oil baths, nasal administrations, and herbal enemas. It is a revitalizing and gratifying experience for both the body and the mind. *Panchakarma* is a common treatment recommended by Ayurveda for maintaining proper personal health and mental equilibrium. It is also referred to as a five-fold treatment. It is tailored to each person based on their specific requirements. It varies greatly and is determined by the individual's Ayurvedic constitutional form, *dosh*ic imbalances, maturity, gastrointestinal ability, and immune strength (Lad, 2002).

5

FINALLY, YOU ARE PREGNANT!

According to the Ayurvedic text *Charaka Samhita*, *shukra* (sperm) is secreted when a man has intercourse with a *rutumati* woman (a woman who is in her ovulatory stage of the menstrual cycle). This reaches the uterus through the proper passage (vagina) and combines with *aartava* (*streebija*). Due to the connection of *satva* (mind), *jivatma* (spirit) appears in the *garbha* at this period (zygote). This *garbha* (fetus) develops normally and is delivered at the right time. Throughout this period, the mother-to-be's diet must be high in nutrition and be aimed toward the nourishment of not one but two lives (Pashte, 2017).

Although pregnancy tests and ultrasounds are the only certain ways to find out whether you are pregnant, there are other signs and symptoms that you can be aware of. For instance, if you have missed more than one period, it may be a sign that you are pregnant. Signs include morning sickness, sensitivity to smells, and exhaustion.

The first week of pregnancy is determined by the date of your last menstrual cycle. Even if you weren't pregnant at the time, your last menstrual cycle is considered week one of pregnancy. The first day of your last period is used as a measure of the due date. In this section, we will talk about early signs that you may be pregnant.

Cramping and Spotting: From the first to the fourth week, all body changes will happen at a cellular level. The fertilized egg makes a blastocyst (a group of cells filled with fluid). The blastocyst will eventually develop into the baby's organs and body parts. At the 10–14-day mark after pregnancy, the blastocyst implants itself on the lining of the uterus. This can cause light bleeding, which is often mistaken for a period. It is one of the earliest signs that you are pregnant. Look at the color of the blood: in cases of spotting, the color of the blood may be pink or red or brown. If it is spotting, blood will only appear when you wipe the area, rather than in a constant flow. The bleeding usually lasts three days or less.

Fatigue: While fatigue can occur at any point, during the pregnancy, it is also one of the earliest signs that you may be pregnant. This is the result of your progesterone levels rising high, the natural consequence of which is to feel sleepier.

Palpitations: Your heart can begin to beat faster and harder around the eighth week or up to week 10. During pregnancy, palpitations and arrhythmias are normal. The blood flow in the body increases during pregnancy. To circulate the extra blood, the heart must pump harder, which can result in a faster resting heart rate. The extra strain on the heart can often cause palpitations.

Tingling, Aching, or Increase in Breast Size: Between the fourth and sixth weeks, breast changes are probable. Due to hormonal changes, you are more likely to grow tender and swollen breasts. This should subside after a few weeks as the body adjusts to the hormones.

About week 11, nipple and breast adjustments are also possible. Hormones continue to cause breast development. The areola – the area around the nipple – can darken and grow in size.

If you had acne before becoming pregnant, you may experience a pregnancy-induced breakout again. This is not a permanent outcome of pregnancy, so you do not need to worry.

Mood Changes: During pregnancy, the estrogen and progesterone levels will be elevated. This increase can influence your mood, making you more emotional or reactive than normal. Mood swings are normal during pregnancy and may lead to depression, restlessness, agitation, or elation.

Frequent Urination: Your body increases the amount of blood it pumps during pregnancy. As a result, the kidney processes more fluid than normal, resulting in more fluid in your bladder.

Hormones play an important role in bladder health as well. You may find yourself needing to use the restroom more often or inadvertently leaking. Please do not feel embarrassed by this because it is completely natural.

Constipation and Bloating: Progesterone relaxes muscles in your body, and your body releases more progesterone to sustain your pregnancy. This includes the intestinal muscles. Slower moving intestine muscles indicate a slowing of digestion. This causes gas to accumulate, resulting in bloating, burping, and flatulence.

Nausea and Morning Sickness: Nausea and morning sickness normally appear between the fourth and sixth weeks. While it is referred to as morning sickness, it can occur at any time of day or night. The exact cause of nausea and morning sickness is unknown, but hormones may contribute. Many women experience moderate to serious morning sickness during their first trimester. It may become more serious toward the end of the first trimester, but it usually subsides when you reach the second trimester.

Smell Aversion to Certain Food Items: Smell sensitivity is a common early pregnancy symptom that is mostly self-diagnosed. There is no scientific evidence that scent aversion occurs during the first trimester of pregnancy. However, it may be significant because smell exposure may cause nausea and vomiting. It can also induce a deep aversion to some foods.

Weight Gain: Gaining weight becomes more normal at the end of the first trimester. You can gain between one and four pounds in the first few months. The calorie requirements for early pregnancy will be similar to your regular diet, but they will rise as the pregnancy progresses.

Pregnancy Glow: Many people may begin to refer to you as having the "pregnancy glow." More blood flows into the vessels because of increased blood volume and higher hormone levels. As a result, the body's oil glands work extra hard, making your skin shine!

THE DIFFERENT STAGES

Ayurvedic literature mentions the different phases that your baby will go through during the pregnancy. *Kalala,* which is representative of an irregular, tiny form, emerges from the womb as an embryo. Up to the 10th day, it is known as *budbuda*. This denotes blastocyst formation, which starts about the fifth day. By the 15th day, it becomes *ghana* (solid). Up to the 20th day, it transforms into a lump of flesh (*mamsapinda*). By the 25th day, *panchamahabhuta maka,* or organ development, begins (Pashte, 2017).

By your second month of pregnancy, the child's sex can be predicted. If a solid mass is oval in shape (*pinda*), the child is male; and if it is elongated (*peshi*), the child is female. According to Ayurvedic texts, by the 50th day, the budlike structure of future body parts is created (*garbhankura*). The development of body parts becomes visible in the third month. Five buds, that is, one for the head and four for the upper and lower extremities, become more and more apparent. At this stage, the embryo begins to develop consciousness and is receptive to feelings like pain (Pashte, 2017).

By the fourth month, different body parts take coherent shape, and the fetus becomes stable. Consciousness and the beating of the heart are more apparent. The fetus begins understanding the need to nourish itself, and at this stage, the character and behavior of the future child can be adjusted depending on the taste of the food items the mother wishes to consume. In the fifth month, the fetus begins to develop mental consciousness and viability. The sixth month is marked by a solidification of the fetus's intelligence. This month emphasizes the growth of hair, nails, bone, tendons, and the accumulation of energy and skin complexion and health. During the seventh month, all organs and body parts are properly formed. There is a danger of instability of *ojas* in the eighth month, so Ayurvedic texts advise that the mother should be careful during this time (Pashte, 2017). The ninth month is marked by giving birth.

How Ayurveda Looks at Your Pregnancy

Most contemporary medical recommendations for the mother-to-be will simply tell them to avoid alcohol, smoking, drugs, and excess physical exertion. Ayurveda, on the other hand, treats pregnancy with special care and nourishment and attempts to nurture the mother and the fetus during the whole period. It tries to ensure proper growth and development of the fetus, adequate secretion of breast milk, and a pregnancy where the mother or her child does not suffer the effects of a poor diet like anemia. A diet which ensures all these conditions allows for a safe and wholesome pregnancy and childbirth.

The *apana vata* must be kept in balance during your pregnancy. It controls the body's upward and downward motions and is primarily found in the colon, large intestine, rectum, pelvic cavity, vagina and cervix, kidneys, urinary tract, prostrate, scrotum, testes, and penis. It is commonly found in organs ranging from the navel to the pelvic floor. Though all three *doshas* (*vata*, *pitta*, and *kapha*) must be balanced during pregnancy, *vata* is the most essential in ensuring a healthy pregnancy. *Apana vata* influences the growth and development of the fetus and is important for a stable and natural delivery.

There are some signs that can tell you that your *apana vata* has been vitiated. These include regular indigestion, constipation, urine retention/painful passage of urine, back pain, infections in the anal rectal tract, bone weakness, exhaustion, and low sex drive. Ayurveda suggests the use of some herbs to restore balance to your *apana vata*. While we shall discuss them, it is advisable for you to consult a specialist before you begin any dosage or consumption (Swati, 2021).

Haritaki is a key component of the potent *Triphala*. It has a fantastic effect on *Apana vata* management. It improves digestion and digests any undigested food substances in the system. It has a slightly laxative (purgatory) action that helps to hold the *apana* in check by encouraging its action in the colon, which is one of its primary places. It is also used in many *snigdha virechana* therapies, where it is mixed with castor oil and administered. Except for saltiness, it contains all six tastes according to Ayurveda. It is also rich in anti-aging properties and enhances both longevity and intelligence. Take one or two grams of *haritaki* powder mixed with jaggery on a regular basis.

The root of the Indian valerian plant, known as *tagara* is also thought to be beneficial for balancing vitiated *apana vata*. When *apana* is out of control, the colon produces *ama* (toxins). The mild laxative nature of the plant, together with its *deepana* (digestive fire kindling herbs) and *pachana* (for digesting the ama), calms the *apana vata* and redirects its movement downward. It purifies the intestines and blood. The herb should be used with care because it can aggravate *pitta* and overall acidity; it should be consumed in small amounts only (Swati, 2021).

In Indian households, asafoetida is a common spice. It is a great cure for bloating, gas, distension, and digestive problems. It is also known as *hing*. *Deepena* (digestive), *pachana* (toxin digestive), *krimighna* (anti-parasitic), and *sulaprasamana* (relieves intestinal spasms) are all properties of *hing*. It is especially beneficial for *apana vata* due to its *Anulomana* property. *Anulomana* refers to any herb or medicine that dissolves the obstruction of *malas* (waste) and directs it downward by redirecting the flow of the *apana vata*. This property is extremely beneficial for minimizing bloating (Swati, 2021). To normalize the direction of *apana* flow, take a pinch of *hing* with a glass of warm water. You can also dry roast some *hing* and mix it with buttermilk to achieve the same effect.

Sunthi, or dry Ginger, is known as one of the most effective Ayurvedic herbs for balancing vitiated *vata* in the body. It is an excellent digestive herb for the treatment of *adhman* (bloating), *ajirna* (indigestion), *chhardi* (vomiting), *sula* (stomach pain/colicky pain), *arsha* (hemorrhoids), *agnimandya* (loss of appetite), and other digestive problems. Since it is *grahi* (absorbent) and bowel binding, it is useful in both irritable bowel syndrome and constipation. Usually, pungent-tasting herbs increase *vata*, but *sunthi* and *pippali* are exceptions since they balance *vata*. Consuming three to seven grams of *sunthi* for two months will result in substantial reduction of digestive pain and inflammation.

Ajwain is a spice that is commonly used in Indian kitchens. It is one of the most effective herbs for treating *vata* imbalances in the stomach. It aids in the stimulation of the appetite and the improvement of digestion. When combined with ***kala namak*** (black salt), it relieves gas in a matter of minutes. It has a strong effect on the *apana vata* in the lower pelvic area, which houses the sexual organs. It increases libido by improving sperm secretion and regulating sexual hormones. It is also a mild laxative and directs the *apana vata* in the correct downward direction (Swati, 2021).

In general, you can balance vitiated *dosha* by following some specific steps:

- Consume a *vata*-balancing diet.
- Wear clothing that is not too tight in the abdominal and/or pelvic region. This interrupts the flow of *apana*.
- Light exercise and yoga will help you break free from a sedentary lifestyle.
- To monitor vitiated *vata*, perform an *abhyanga* (oil massage) with sesame oil before taking a warm water bath.
- Cook with warm spices such as cinnamon, black pepper, cumin, fennel, ginger, and cloves.
- Avoid being exposed to cold weather.

You may be wondering if there are any tips for balancing your diet to ensure proper flow of *apana vata*. The good news is that you don't need to go overboard! Simple home remedies will help you keep your *vata* in balance.

You can soak a handful of raisins, two to three figs, and two prunes overnight and consume them in the mornings. Buttermilk is a great digestive drink, and you can use this as a refreshing accompaniment to all your meals. It will work wonders for you, unlike pop and fizzy sodas. If you are not lactose intolerant, you can consume clarified butter (*ghee*) and milk. Coconut milk is also a good option. Avoid consuming any leftovers. The food you eat should be rich in freshness, or *prana.* The longer cooked food remains unconsumed, the more it loses its *prana*. Go for lentils that are easier to digest, such as black lentils and French green lentils. Finally, avoid excessive consumption of starchy food items like potatoes ("Prana in Food," 2017).

A diet that is primarily sweet, liquid, cooling, and easy to digest is ideal for a pregnant woman. During the first three months of pregnancy, the primary goal is to keep the fetus alive. The mother's diet must ensure that the fetus stays healthy and that there is no vaginal bleeding. The fetus grows and develops at its fastest from the fourth to the seventh month. This is made possible by the diet during this period. At the final stage, the mother must be prepared to endure the pressure of a regular delivery. The mother's diet and treatment are intended to facilitate this. Sweet foods are recommended during this period because they provide the body with the most nourishment and development.

Some naturally sweet food items include sweet fruits like mangos, coconut, berries, and bananas, and dry fruits like raisins and figs.

Vegetables like beets, carrots, zucchini, and pumpkins are good for consumption during pregnancy. Rice and wheat can be consumed. Jaggery and honey are good condiments to sweeten your food with. Mung beans and red lentils are cooling and therefore good sources of protein; dairy and tofu can also be consumed. Finally, spices and condiments like cardamom, cinnamon, vanilla, saffron, coriander, and bay leaf are all great additions to the diet of a pregnant woman ("Naturally Sweet Foods: The Most Satvik Of All As Per Ayurveda," 2019).

As a mother-to-be, avoid situations that make you angry, incite fear or terror, aggravate you, or cause emotional trauma. Do not expose yourself to any jealousy. Do not indulge in excessively hard physical activity, carry heavy loads, or do anything that will cause undue strain to your body. Do not indulge in sights or shows which are too violent or unpleasant – remember that everything has a cognitive imprint. Do not show undue anger or abuse. Travel in comfortable vehicles. Make sure to get a minimum of eight hours of sleep in a day. Engage in light to moderate physical activity, particularly exercises that will strengthen your pelvic floor. Finally, try to maintain a conscious balance of the different *doshas* and take good care of your diet at all times.

6

MONTHLY DIET SUPPLEMENTS

As you proceed with your pregnancy, you must look at ways to ensure that your diet is healthy, nourishing, and capable of strengthening both you and your baby. To allow for this, Ayurveda makes room for diet supplements in every month of your pregnancy. These are not pills that may have chemical side effects on your body, rather, they are remedies drawn from and dependent upon nature, and they will work to enhance your and your unborn baby's health. These are herbs and plants that grow in nature. The beauty of Ayurveda is that it believes nature has all the remedies that your body needs to stay happy and healthy.

Month One: Milk is an essential part of the diet throughout the first month of your pregnancy. Whenever you consume milk, ensure that it is at room temperature. You can enhance its cooling effect by using *bala* to process it. *Bala* is a plant that can be found growing wild in open areas. It is especially helpful during pregnancy. It has a cooling effect on your stomach and a sweet flavor. It provides strength and enhances the appearance of the skin, and it is of a fatty nature (Girija, 2013). *Bala*, like milk, helps to avoid bleeding. It is a great herb for calming *pitta* and controlling *vayu*.

During this month, you should aim for a cooling, sweet, and liquid diet. Examples could include rice with milk taken two times a day. This meal should also protect you from bleeding. Do not rub or massage the body with oils or medicinal concoctions at this time.

Month Two: In the second month, you can make a decoction of milk by boiling it with medicinal herbs, straining and cooling, and then drinking it. Herbs that are commonly prescribed at this time include *bala, shatavari,* and *yashti. Yashti* has a cooling effect, is sweet in taste, and is good for your skin and body strength. It has an oily nature and can also be beneficial for your hair's health. It is known to control *pitta* and *vata. Shatavari* is a special herb that has a mildly bitter taste. It has a cooling effect and is sweet. It rejuvenates your body, improves your digestive capacity, and increases strength. It controls and balances *pitta* (Girija, 2013).

You can take a cup of milk, mix it with ½ cup of water and 50 grams of the herb, and boil this until the water evaporates. Strain the milk and let it cool completely before you consume it. You can add a little sugar if you wish to make it sweeter. Your diet should preferably be liquid during this month.

Month Three: Nausea and vomiting are the most noticeable and frequent symptoms in the early stages of pregnancy. This causes a lot of pain for some women. About the third month, it normally starts to bother them. This month's diet aids them in overcoming this problem. For a pregnant woman in her third month, honey mixed with milk and *ghee* (all at room temperature) is recommended (Girija, 2013).

Honey is only recommended during the third month of pregnancy. It has a non-greasy (dry) texture and a sweet, slightly astringent flavor. It is thought to be the most effective treatment for *kapha*. Honey improves vision, quenches appetite, and prevents bleeding (including pre-term bleeding in pregnancy) and vomiting. However, be careful with how you are consuming it. Honey should never be heated before consumption. Do not consume in large amounts because it will lead to indigestion.

During this month, the recommended diet is rice porridge (*kanji*) with milk.

If you are experiencing extreme bouts of discomfort and vomiting, you can try some natural remedies. These include:

- *Dhaniya* (coriander) paste mixed with a thin rice gruel and sugar
- A soup made with green gram and pomegranate seeds, salt, and *ghee*

- A soup made of goat meat without salt, soured with pomegranate, and seasoned with tasty spices such as ginger, pepper, cinnamon, and cardamom. This relieves vomiting, especially vomiting induced by *vayu* aggravation.
- Rice gruel mixed with sugar, honey, and spices such as cardamom, cinnamon, and cloves is particularly effective in treating vomiting caused by *pitta* aggravation.
- A decoction of sweet mango and *jamun* (black plum) mixed with honey is effective in treating vomiting caused by *kapha* aggravation (phlegm).

These are natural remedies that do not have any side effects. You can use combinations of these depending on the levels of your discomfort and appetite.

Month Four: During this month, all the body parts of the fetus have begun taking shape. A diet that is rich in butter extracted from milk is beneficial at this time. Around a tablespoon of butter can be added to a glass of milk (around a cup). The butter that is extracted directly from milk is known as *navaneeta*. It is a fatty substance that is sweet in taste. It has a cooling effect and prevents premature bleeding. It also aids digestion and is beneficial for the skin. It cures imbalances of *vata* and *pitta* (Girija, 2013).

During this month, you can consume a soup made from meat. The meat should not be fatty. During pregnancy, frequent use of meat is not recommended since it is very heavy on your stomach. At this time, however, consuming this soup can help in nourishing your fetus.

Month Five: During this month, consumption of clarified butter or *ghee* is encouraged. You can add *ghee* to milk porridge and enhance the flavor of a light meat broth with it. It is beneficial to those suffering from herpes, or those with *vata* and *pitta* imbalances. It can heal and nourish your body. It has a cooling effect, and when mixed with other substances, it can take on the quality of those substances without losing its own potency (Girija, 2013).

Month Six: During this month, rice gruel, *ghee* processed with sweet herbs, and *gokshura* comprise an ideal diet. This diet acts against fluid retention in your body. It cools, strengthens and nourishes you while also balancing your *vata*.

Gokshura is a cooling and strengthening herb for the body. It has a nice flavor and aids in digestion. One of the most essential properties of *gokshura* is that it is an outstanding treatment for all urinary system disorders. It cleanses the urinary system, makes urination easier, eliminates urinary stones, and regulates diabetes. It can help with respiratory issues, cough, piles, and heart disease. It balances the body's irritated *vayu*.

Month Seven: The diet of this month is basically the same as the other six months, but a plant that is used for this specific month is the *vidari* plant. At this time, *vidari*-processed *ghee* is an excellent supplement. *Vidari* is rich in medicinal properties and is particularly beneficial to expectant mothers. It has a sweet taste and a cooling effect. Its properties are fatty, high in nourishment, and it provides strength to the body. *Vidari* reduces inflammation and balances *vata* and *pitta*. It is helpful for curing any disorders of the blood.

This month may be accompanied by some skin issues like rashes and burning sensations. This can be the result of an imbalance of the *doshas* which get pushed up to the chest because of the growing fetus and cause itching and burning. You should not scratch or damage your skin. If the itching becomes too much, make a paste of sandalwood, and apply it to the affected areas. Avoid salt and oil as much as you can. Stay hydrated and consume food items that will pacify your *vata*.

Month Eight: The main goal of the last two months of your pregnancy is to prepare you for your impending delivery. A thin gruel fortified with milk and *ghee* is the best meal for a pregnant woman during the eighth month. This benefits the mother's health while still nourishing the fetus. During this month, you can take two medicated enemas or *vastis* (a medicinal decoction enema accompanied by a medicated oil enema) to help you prepare for a smooth delivery (Girija, 2013).

Month Nine: Food mixed with *ghee* and meat soup, or thick gruel mixed with fat, preferably *ghee*, is ideal for you during the ninth month. This ensures that you are safe and strong enough to deliver the baby. During this month, you can take a medicated oil enema. This will stabilize your bowel movements and balance your *vata*, preparing you for a natural, relaxed delivery (Girija, 2013).

Tips

Before we move on, here are two tips that can give you some additional help in these nine beautiful months!

- The use of *dhanvantara tailam* is recommended during pregnancy. This oil, also known as *bala dhanvantara tailam*, is made up of over forty ingredients, the most important of which is *bala*. *Dhanvantara tailam* is beneficial in the treatment of all *vata* diseases; it cures diseases of women after childbirth and diseases of children; it is beneficial to people suffering from injuries (*marma*) and bone defects; and it is beneficial to people who are emaciated or have problems like anemia. It also assists in the treatment of genital tract disorders and can help cure certain fevers, abdominal tumors, and psychological illnesses.
- Excessive consumption of yogurt should be avoided by women, particularly during pregnancy. It is warming (in terms of efficacy) and can increase bleeding and may cause premature bleeding. Yogurt can also make you bloat. As a result, consuming too much of it during pregnancy causes the body to retain excess fluid.

The supplements and meals which are recommended for you during your pregnancy, from the start to the end, work toward helping you prepare for normal childbirth. They soften your uterus, strengthen your pelvis, and make your reproductive system malleable. They aid your bowel movements, ease body pain, and help in the downward flow of *vayu*, which is essential for childbirth (Girija, 2013). Remember that your nutrition must be adequate for two people – you and your baby. Plan your supplements accordingly. However, before you begin any supplements, consult a licensed professional so that you know the best options for you.

LABOR AND CHILDBIRTH

The ninth month begins on the first day of the month and ends on the first day of the 10th month. This is the time frame for a standard delivery. Obstetricians typically look at pregnancy as something that lasts for a period of 280 days beginning on the first day of the previous menstrual cycle. However, a pregnancy that lasts past the "due date" is not uncommon. This does not have to be a cause for concern. From the beginning of the ninth month, delivery can occur on any day, and in some rare cases, pregnancy may continue past the 10th month.

You may feel pain or mild contractions on some days, particularly if you are nearing your due date. These types of pains normally go away on their own. If these pains last too long or are too severe, *vayu*-pacifying home remedies are administered. Some of these remedies include juice squeezed from the leaves of drumstick plants (*Moringa oleifera*), and decoctions made from *saunf* (anise), jaggery, black cumin, and garlic.

As the time for delivery draws close, some women prefer to spend a period in silence and self-observation. If you are one of them, you can consider meditation and self-transformation coaching centers that teach you to reach out to your inner selves. *Vipassana* is one such technique that is revered in countries like India. This looks at the connection between the mind and the body. The only way to experience it is by paying attention to all the physical sensations that construe your life force. It relies on self-exploration and observation and is a 10-day long course that does not allow you to indulge in any speech. You are to remain quiet and meditative during this time. The result is a balanced mind that is rich in understanding, empathy, and love (Goenka, 2021).

So, what does labor really feel like? In simple words, labor is the natural process that your body goes through as it enters the childbirth phase. It begins when your contractions are steady and lasts until the delivery of your baby and placenta. Unfortunately, no one knows exactly what triggers labor or when it will begin, but a number of physical and hormonal changes will help to signal the start of labor.

Just before the start of labor, your baby will lower into your pelvis and settle there. This phenomenon is known as the baby "dropping" into your pelvis. This can happen at any point, between a few hours to a week before you enter labor. You may feel the need to use the washroom more often. Since your upper abdomen is now empty, you will have more room to breathe and may feel relief from heartburn or inflammation, which are common in the early stages of pregnancy. As your cervix begins to open, the mucus plug that accumulates there is discharged into your vagina. This plug may look clear, pink, or may be slightly bloody. Labor can begin soon after this discharge or even one or two weeks later.

The regularity of labor pains may be used to identify it. They appear at regular intervals, and their power gradually builds up. Initially, the time between contractions is about 10 minutes. It decreases over time. The time between two contractions can be as short as one minute near the end. Each contraction will last anywhere from 30 seconds to a minute. It is natural to feel fatigued as labor approaches, and your limbs may ache regardless of physical exercise. You can experience looseness in the belly, as if a knot is being untied from the chest. In some cases, you may feel unusually sleepy, experience loss of taste and appetite, as well as increased salivation and urination. There is pain and discomfort in the legs, belly, waist, back, heart area, bladder, and vagina, as well as vaginal discharge. You may notice a prickling or pulsation in the vaginal region. This sensation is usually followed by the onset of labor pain and discharge of amniotic fluid.

The muscles of the uterus tighten during contractions, and the abdomen becomes rigid. In between these contractions, you will feel your uterus relaxing and the abdomen softening. Each woman's experience with a contraction is unique, and it may vary from one pregnancy to the next. In most cases, labor contractions cause pain or a dull ache in the back and lower abdomen, as well as pressure in the pelvis. Contractions travel in a wave pattern from the top to the bottom of the uterus. You can experience the sensation of a heavy menstrual cramp. True labor contractions, unlike false labor contractions or Braxton Hicks contractions, do not cease when you shift positions or relax. However, you will be able to relax in between contractions, despite how painful they are.

Every woman goes through three stages of labor before childbirth happens. We will discuss each stage briefly.

Stage One/Early and Active Labor: When you start to experience frequent contractions, the cervix opens (dilates), softens, shortens, and thins. This is the first step of labor and birth. This makes it possible for the baby to enter the birth canal. The first stage is the lengthiest of the three. This stage is further divided into early and active labor.

During early labor, the cervix will efface and dilate. You will notice irregular contractions, and they will feel mild. As the cervix begins to open, a discharge will be released from your vagina ("Stages of Labor and Birth: Baby, It's Time!," 2020). This is the mucus plug. The duration of early labor is subject to change. First-time pregnancies can last anywhere from a few hours to a few days. It is not a comfortable time because you can do nothing except wait until the contractions become more frequent and intense. You have to try and stay relaxed. Try going for a walk, taking a cooling shower, listening to some meditative music, practicing relaxation or breathing techniques, or taking a small nap. Be sure that you are not experiencing any complications. If you are experiencing unusually heavy vaginal bleeding, call for help immediately.

During active labor, your cervix will experience a dilation from six centimeters to 10 centimeters. Your contractions will feel stronger, be more closely spaced and occur regularly. You may feel nauseated, and your legs may begin cramping. If your water hasn't already broken, it may do so now, and you may find a heavy pressure building in your back. Now is the time to head to the delivery room. Your pain may grow as labor intensifies. Active labor can often last anywhere between four and eight hours. At this time, your cervix will experience a dilation of about one centimeter each hour. To increase comfort, change your positions, take a cooling shower, practice mindful meditation, and take deep breaths between contractions ("Stages of Labor and Birth: Baby, It's Time!," 2020).

Transition, which occurs at the end of active labor, may be especially severe and painful. Contractions will be close together and will last anywhere between 60 and 90 seconds. Pressure can be felt in your lower back and rectum. If you want to push but aren't completely dilated, your medical professional can advise you to wait. Pushing too early will render you exhausted and cause your cervix to swell, causing delivery to be delayed. Try to pant in between contractions for some relief. Transition takes between 15 to 60 minutes on average.

Stage Two/Birthing Your Baby: During the second stage of labor, you will give birth to your child. Pushing your baby into the world will take anything from a few minutes to several hours or more. For first-time mothers and women who have had an epidural, it can take longer. You will have advice from your healthcare provider on when to push or when to bear down through each contraction. Alternatively, you can be asked to press if you feel the need. When you are pushing, try not to tense up your face. Keep your head down and focus on pushing through the correct spots. Squatting, sitting, kneeling, and even going down on the hands and knees are all viable options for pushing. Try to experiment until you find a position that is right for you.

At some point, you will be asked to push gently or to stop pushing. Slowing down allows the vaginal tissues to stretch instead of tearing. If your baby's head is out, you might ask to feel the baby's head between your legs or see it in a mirror to gain strength and confidence to keep going. Following the delivery of your baby's head, the rest of the baby's body will be delivered soon after. If required, his or her airway will be cleared. The umbilical cord will then be cut by your doctor or labor coach.

Stage Three/Delivering the Placenta: You will probably feel a great sense of relief after your baby is born. Enjoy the moment; however, a lot is still going on. The placenta will be delivered during the third stage of labor. The placenta is usually delivered in five to 30 minutes, but it can take up to an hour. Try to unwind. Your attention has most likely shifted to your child. You could be completely unaware of what's going on around you. Try breastfeeding your baby if you like. Mild contractions will continue to occur, but they will be closer together and much less painful.

You will have to push once more to deliver the placenta, which will then be examined to ensure everything is okay. To avoid bleeding and infection, any remaining fragments must be ultimately removed from the uterus. Your uterus will begin to contract after you deliver the placenta to help it return to its usual size. Your abdomen will be massaged by a member of your health care team to ensure that the uterus is firm. Your doctor will also decide if you need stitches or repair for any vaginal tears. If you don't have anesthesia, a local anesthetic will be injected into the stitching region ("Stages of Labor and Birth: Baby, It's Time!," 2020).

Ayurveda looks at the final stages before giving birth as a time of being surrounded by love and kindness. The mother will want to be surrounded by her female friends and family, while being massaged gently with warmed oil over her back, hips, thighs, and flanks. If there is a problem of labor not progressing, she is told to inhale a *chooram* (powder) made from medicinal herbs. This inhalation can also be given during contractions. The application of medicinal paste around the umbilical cord can aid in labor moving forward.

On the Topic of Circumcision

It is fascinating to see circumcision through the lens of *marma* (energy points similar to acupuncture points) and the *chakras*. Our genital organs are a massive energetic hub with many nerve endings and blood supply. In other words, this part of the body transmits, receives and exudes a lot of energy. While the male penis has many vital *marma* or energy points, the *medhra marma* point, which is the most important, is located at the tip of the penis. During the circumcision process, this point is subject to direct manipulation. This point is crucial not just for sexual energy but also for the stimulation of *ojas*, the essence of vitality and immunity in our bodies.

Mishandling this specific point can result in serious health consequences.

Consider the second *chakra* from the root, the *swadhisthana* chakra. The unconscious, thoughts, and desires are all connected to this *chakra*. It is connected to the reproductive organs in the body. According to *chakra* therapy and theory, inappropriate manipulation of a *chakra* and its associated organs will result in a blockage of *prana* in that *chakra*. Emotional instability and relationship problems, as well as difficulties with creativity, can arise in this situation (Devani, 2016).

Ultimately, the decision regarding circumcision rests in your hands. If you choose to circumcise, you can do some things to ease the whole process. Following the circumcision, try to provide the baby with an anti-*vata* surrounding that is enveloped in love and security. Your warmth and a warm temperature are the most important things you can provide to your baby at that moment. Consider breastfeeding your baby because this creates a beautiful bonding between the mother and the child. Massage your baby with warm oil daily. Once the incision has healed, press on the *medhra marma* point as gently as possible so as to support the *ojas*.

This is the stage where you get to breathe and revel in all the work that you have put in for the last nine months. The evidence of how much your body is capable of rests in your arms.

Congratulations, you are now a mother! As we move on, let us look at some things that you can do to enhance your own postpartum recovery.

8

POSTPARTUM RECOVERY

Following childbirth, as a new mother, you need special attention and diligence. If you contract a disease soon after giving birth, it may quickly progress to a severe or incurable condition. During pregnancy, the nourishment you acquire is needed to help in the growth and overall development of the fetus. As a result, all of your body's *dhatus* (such as *rasa*, blood, and so on) are diminished and weakened. Your health is fragile due to the strains of labor and the loss of fluid and blood during childbirth, as well as the emptiness produced in the body after childbirth. To replenish and revitalize yourself, Ayurvedic literature prescribes a diet with the aim of increasing your immunity and preventing you from contracting diseases.

A mixture of *ghee* and oil is massaged onto your body after you have given birth and then bathed in warm decoctions made from herbs that calm *vata*. You can take baths in this manner in the morning and evening, which relieves the stress and pressure of the delivery. An empty space is formed after delivery in your abdomen. A cloth can be wrapped around your abdomen for a few days to prevent *vata* from entering the empty space and causing abdominal inflammation and other disorders.

You should be provided medicines and a special diet that is sweet in flavor and provides strength, good nutrition, and immunity from *vata* ailments. In the first week, only food items that are light on your stomach and easily digestible should be consumed. Heavy and rich food should be introduced only after a week of light meals. You can consume meat and fish after 12 days. Fermented preparations can be introduced in your diet because they heal the uterus and encourage the production of breast milk.

Food items processed with medicinal herbs are needed for you to recuperate from your postpartum status. They help enhance your psychological and physical health, nourish your body, and balance your *dhatus*. A miracle worker at this time is *Sowbhagya Sunthi*. It is a traditional formulation from the Ayurvedic text *Rasa Ratna Samuccaya*. *Sowbhagya Sunthi* is a medicinal compound made from a combination of herbs. It gets its name from one of its key ingredients, dry ginger (*sunthi*). It is given to women after they have given birth. Fever, liver and spleen disorders, constipation, anemia, abdominal tumors, loss of appetite, cough, respiratory diseases, worms, and poor digestion are all treated with *Sowbhagya Sunthi*.

You can introduce it into your daily diet to improve your overall health and nourishment.

The process of childbirth leaves an empty space inside the womb, allowing air to fill it and causing an imbalance in the *vata* force. Anxiety, dryness, gas, constipation, bloating, and disturbed sleep are all symptoms of this. The aim of Ayurvedic postpartum treatment is to balance your *vata*. After childbirth, Ayurveda recognizes the importance of taking care of the mother and works to balance the *vata dosha* for 42 days (or six weeks). Calming *vata*, alleviating *vayu*, and promoting physical and psychological well-being are all important aspects of postpartum treatment designed for restoring your wellbeing. After losing energy, blood, and fluids, not to mention the creation of a large amount of room in the abdomen, you are full of mobile, light, dry, and cold qualities (previously occupied by the baby). When you add in the sleep deprivation and exhaustion that comes with feeding and nourishing an infant, it is easy to see how your body will feel disjointed and out of balance.

You will know your *vata* is out of balance if you have bouts of anxiety, fear and panic. Your body or body parts will be prone to spasms and twitches. Your skin can become drier, you can experience bloating, constipation, and lose body weight. You will feel more sensitive to the cold and to wind, and you will have trouble hearing loud noises. Your sleep will become disturbed, and you may feel scattered, like your mind is in a thousand different places. At this point, your focus should be on a diet of food items that will alleviate your *vata dosha*. You can consume tofu, tempeh, soy milk at room temperature, and some legumes like split green beans. You can treat your liquid items with cinnamon and nutmeg. Spices like ginger, cinnamon, cumin, and black pepper are good for pacifying *vata*. Add a good amount of *ghee* to your diet. Avoid consuming carbonated drinks or too much alcohol. Try not to overeat and try avoiding deep-fried food items.

To restore your balance in the first few weeks after postpartum, there are certain remedies that you can follow.

First, take adequate rest. You are advised to spend time resting at home for 40 days (six weeks) so that you do not come in touch with external influences that can adversely affect you or your baby's health. It is common to seek rest and shelter in your parental homes following pregnancy or for your guardians to come and help with the baby and other household tasks including cooking and cleaning. This is absolutely fine, but beyond this, avoid any influences that will incite excitement or too much passion in you. New motherhood is exhausting, and it is natural for you to feel tired and overwhelmed, so take time out to rest and simply be with your baby and yourself.

An access point for air to the body is said to be the nose and the ears. Many health care providers recommend that pregnant women (and new mothers) cover their ears with cotton to avoid fluctuations in the *vata dosha*. Keeping feet warm is a natural way to balance *vata* as well. Securing a balance in your *vata* is also one of the reasons why the new mother's abdomen is surgically tied during the period immediately after delivery: to keep it from being stretched out and to prevent excess gas from entering.

The connection between your baby and you is unbreakable, and any stimuli that you experience when you are pregnant can have an effect on your baby. Due to this, pregnant women and new mothers should always surround themselves with positive influences and environments. Watch happy television shows, read positive books, and indulge in good memories and events. Surround yourself with a soothing environment filled with fulfilling thoughts which will make you feel uplifted, particularly when you are breastfeeding.

You should consume properly prepared soft and digestible foods that are easily digested. These will aid in the regulation of *vata* and replenish *agni* (the digestive fire). Prepare your meals with *ghee*. The main function of *ghee* is to support digestion and to help make food energy levels remain stable and encourage bowel movements. Also, foods which are rich in herbs and spices will help relieve flatulence and boost your milk supply (Chimnani, 2021a).

Avoid vegetables like cauliflower, chickpeas, and beans because these cause bloating and gas. Some communities encourage the consumption of meaty broths, bone marrow soups, and warm milk. Your baby will also be nursing frequently, and this can be exhausting. Snack on food items that are rich in Omega-3 fatty acids, which are typically available in most kinds of nuts. You are encouraged to sip on warm water and consume warm teas so that you stay hydrated. The teas can be a decoction of herbs that will encourage milk production, known as *galactogogues.* This includes fenugreek seeds (*methi*), fennel seeds (*saunf*), cumin seeds (*jeera*), caraway seeds (*ajwain*), and *shatavari*. Other than herbs, *galactogogues* are also found in whole grains like oatmeal.

Ashwagandha tea is an excellent drink to consume at this time. To prepare this tea, boil a cup of water and add a teaspoon of dried ashwagandha root powder to it. Turn the heat down and cover the water with a lid. Allow it to cook on a gentle flame for 10–15 minutes. After 15 minutes, pour into a glass jar with a strainer, and add a teaspoon of turmeric, agave nectar or honey, and cinnamon. Enjoy every sip of this mindfully because it will not only nourish you but work wonders for your body (Chimnani, 2021a).

Another great supplement for this time is golden milk or turmeric milk. To make it, simply add one teaspoon of turmeric paste or powder to hot milk, along with one teaspoon of sugar. Allow this to come down to room temperature before you consume it. Turmeric milk has anti-inflammatory properties that work really well to pacify your *vata*. It also helps unclog milk ducts and heals swollen breast tissues, both of which are beneficial at the time of breastfeeding.

Another important way to restore *vata*'s balance in your body is through oil massages. If your delivery has been uncomplicated, you can start stomach binding and oil massages in the first week of postpartum. If you have had a difficult delivery, begin massages at the close of week two. Take the advice of your health professionals before you begin any massage routine. An experienced massage therapist should be involved in the first three months after delivery, and they will provide you with daily oil massages, also known as *abhyanga.* This will not only heal your body but also nourish your skin.

The therapists will use warm oils that will help in reducing *vata.* These oils are generally infused with herbs like *chandana, ashwagandha, bala,* and *kushta.* They may also contain *eranda* (castor) and *til* (sesame). Olive oil mixed with cloves can also be used for lower back pain. Oil massages are performed in a warm space with the air conditioning turned off and the windows closed to prevent excess air from entering. Sweat is another advantage of being in a warm environment; it is thought to be a safe way for the body to get rid of extra fluids gained during pregnancy (Chimnani, 2021b).

To relieve aching bones and improve circulation, the massage will last up to an hour and is very vigorous. A full body and head massage is normally performed, with extra oil being added to the naval area. Breasts are normally avoided, and the belly is massaged vigorously (if your health allows for it). This, according to Ayurveda, aids in the contraction of the uterus and the return of the organs to their original places. The Ayurveda therapist should be well-versed about the practices behind postpartum diets, healthy parenting, and wholesome motherhood. She should be able to give you emotional support and dispel your suspicions.

A warm oil massage is beneficial for a number of reasons:

- It results in relief from the physical pain that follows a delivery.
- It soothes aches that happen from bearing the weight of a baby all the time. This can be particularly stressful on your shoulders, back, and arms.
- It rejuvenates you and removes your fatigue.
- It strengthens abdominal muscles that may have stretched during the pregnancy and delivery.
- Stability and balance become better with oil massages. They

increase circulation and encourage the flow of blood to different parts of the body.
- Your skin becomes soft and supple, and dryness and itchiness are reduced.
- Most importantly, oil massages provide an overall sense of relaxation and help you regain your natural balance in the environment. You will be able to sleep better and feel rejuvenated. This may in turn induce better lactation.

Your newborn baby can also be involved in the process. They can receive a 15-minute massage daily. This can be done with Ayurvedic or baby oils, depending on what is better for the fragile, sensitive skin of the baby. Extra oil should be gently massaged onto the baby's crown (the slight dip of their head) and their naval areas.

As a matter of fact, you can also indulge in massages with your baby yourself! This will not only increase the bond between the two of you but also result in better health. There are a variety of credible resources online for self-massage, or you can seek professional advice. There are several programs and local classes that teach mothers how to massage their babies, which can be a wonderful way to strengthen the connection between mother and child.

If you get a massage from a therapist, take a warm shower after it. At this time, the massage therapist can give the baby a massage before gently bathing them in warm water. You should have a snack to boost your energy at this stage, such as nuts, protein-rich fox nuts, or nut-based sweetmeats, and then nurse your baby. The warm shower and breast milk will most likely bring the baby to sleep, allowing the massage therapist to concentrate on binding your belly (Chimnani, 2021b). In Ayurveda, the abdomen is bound for 12 hours or overnight with a long muslin or pure cotton cloth. This is to prevent air from entering the uterus and to bring your *vata* into balance. Stomach binding is thought to assist the uterus in contracting, guiding the organs back to their original positions, and providing back support.

Ayurveda provides order and routine to the postpartum cycle through its balanced principles. Each technique has several advantages, both short and long term. It is no surprise that Ayurvedic postpartum treatment is known as "40 days for 40 years" (Chimnani, 2021b). Your recovery will only take some time, but the benefits will last forever.

ON THE TOPIC OF POSTPARTUM DEPRESSION

Childbirth (and pregnancy) is a life-changing experience for both the body and the mind. How a new mother spends the weeks following the birth of her child sets the tone for how the family will work for several years to come. The first 42 days after childbirth were designated by Ayurvedic texts as a time for rest, reinvigoration, and intimacy. In today's world, few mothers have the time or resources to carry out this vital activity. With so much change in new parents' lives, taking this time seems impossible. Unfortunately, the desire to return to "normalcy" has resulted in a variety of physical and emotional postpartum problems that have a long-term negative impact on the woman and her family. Postpartum depression is the most serious problem that women face because of this. Women who suffer from postpartum depression frequently find it difficult to bond with their babies, and many feel shame and guilt even after they have healed (Lewin, 2018).

A mother's first priorities should be bonding with her newborn and relaxing, so a postpartum healing plan should be deliberately easy. Herbs and simple habits will help you achieve your goals and build a solid base for your new family. As a new mother, you may find days where you are depressed, and your mind is scattered. Postpartum depression involves a heady mix of emotional, psychological, behavioral, and physical changes that take over some women after they give birth. It can set in within the first month after the delivery. There are several factors responsible for postpartum depression, including cognitive, social, and chemical changes that happen after you've had your baby.

The overwhelming sensation can become too much to handle, and if left to your devices, this may transition into major depression. The chemical changes occur due to a rapid fall in hormones following delivery. The levels of progesterone and estrogen (your reproductive hormones) can increase 10 times when you are pregnant. Naturally, they fall sharply once you have given birth. They have to return to what they were before you were pregnant, and this can cause a debilitating, disorientating sensation. Handling this depression is something that will need focus, conscious effort, and a lot of time. You have to make room for a lot of acceptance.

Choose to accept yourself as you are. Believe that everything is happening because it is meant to, and there is a purpose behind all of it, even if you cannot immediately grasp that. Make an effort to find happiness and to care for and love yourself as you are, along with your perceived issues and flaws. Question your heart and your mind. Be aware of your emotions, and whenever you find that you are engaging in negative thoughts, such as "Oh, I don't deserve anything/This is useless/My life is meaningless," stop and think of positive things. You have brought new life into this planet. Your worth is more than you can fathom.

Learn to say "no" to things that make you uncomfortable. This will allow you to be responsible for your decisions. If you make choices that go against your comfort or identity, you will feel dissatisfied with their outcomes. To prevent that, say "yes" only when you are certain that you wish to do the activity in question. This is easier said than done, but practice and self-belief are key tactics that will get you there. Without challenges, you cannot grow as you are intended to, so take this as a challenge and practice being assertive about your feelings and choices (Budd, 2020).

Look at the self as a whole. All your negative parts have their own positive aspects. For instance, if you are someone who keeps thinking you aren't good enough, that is tied to a desire to do better. This is not a bad desire in itself – it becomes so because you use it to overexert yourself. The next time you catch yourself thinking this, tell yourself something along the lines of, "I will try to do better when I am feeling good. For now, I will rest." This allows you to transform a negative affirmation into something that is positive and hope-inducing.

Depression is commonly thought of as a *kapha* imbalance in Ayurvedic terms because it includes heaviness, sorrow, and overall stagnation. The official criteria used to diagnose depression include apathy, low energy, a bad mood, and restricted movement. These are all *kapha* issues, indicating that the *kapha dosha* is out of control in the majority of clinical depression cases. From an Ayurvedic perspective, there are three slightly different forms of depression, each referring to one of the three *doshas*. These specific types of depression can affect people with the same primary *dosha*. They can also affect people who have the affected *dosha*(s) out of control, even though they are of a different primary *dosha*.

Kapha depression is predominantly characterized by lethargy, exhaustion, sleepiness, lack of motivation, a feeling of listlessness, and the accumulation of toxins (*ama*) in the body. It is the most common kind of depression, and it tends to last a long time because of the inherently slow nature of *kapha*. Treating *kapha* depression varies but the general ideas are the same – you need to move around more, try to reduce the toxins in your body and the surrounding environment, and center in on your vitality (Budd, 2020). Some recommendations include:

- Practicing yoga every day, particularly *Surya Namaskara* or Sun Salutations.
- Taking 30 minutes of outdoor exercise like walking in nature.
- Increasing the intake of fresh vegetables and reducing consumption of processed and fried food items.
- Eating warm, spicy food and avoiding cold food. Pungent, warming herbs like cinnamon can do wonders for curing *kapha* depression.
- Avoid alcohol.
- Consume ginger tea in the morning and evening.

- Take 300–400 mg *ashwagandha* powder two times a day (morning and evening).
- Consume seaweed like nori and wakame to help boost your metabolism, body temperature, and energy, therefore reducing depression.
- Consume 20–30 mg saffron every day, but make sure to do this after consulting with your physicians, particularly if you are on any other medications.
- Practicing *abhyanga* with a massage therapist and also indulging in self-massages with warm oil will help reduce cortisol and increase serotonin, which make them helpful for curing depression.
- Consume 120–250 mg of *Rhodiola rosea* in the morning, with prior consent of your physicians.
- Consider taking 500 mg of cardamom, which you can add to your tea. Cardamom helps heal inflammation, congestion, and mucus in the body. It also soothes an irritated digestive system. When you feel better physically, your mind automatically responds.
- Avoid long sedentary activities like binge watching television or spending hours on the internet, as these allow *kapha* to accumulate.
- Finally, do simple housework like cleaning the bed. Take calming baths and dress yourself daily. Interact with your close family members so that your vitality is enhanced.

Pitta depression is a more agitated condition. Frustration, indignation, irritability, and impulsivity are common symptoms. Due to the impulsivity and anxiety, this form of depression has a higher risk of suicide. This is known as a "mixed disorder" (depression with manic or psychotic symptoms) or an "agitated depression" in conventional psychiatry. This syndrome is more common in people who have been diagnosed with bipolar disorder or who have any bipolar tendencies (Budd, 2020).

- Engage in slow, restorative yoga for 20 to 30 minutes every day. Hot yoga and strenuous exercise should be avoided.
- Practice meditation every day for 20 minutes, preferably under a tree in nature.
- Practice 30–60 minutes a day, preferably by the ocean, a lake, or a sea. *Pitta* likes water because it is refreshing.
- Alkalinity can be increased in the body by drinking green tea, eating salads, and eating fresh vegetables.
- Increase the intake of cooling foods.
- Spicy foods can cause *pitta* imbalances, so avoid them.
- During the healing process, stay away from alcohol (and be mindful afterward). Alcohol is acidic, which makes *pitta* worse.
- *Pitta* will benefit from aloe vera juice. Cooling and anti-inflammatory, one cup or more a day is recommended. Inflammation is a factor in many cases of depression.
- *Shatavari* is an herb that can be taken in doses of 400–800 mg per day (*Asparagus racemosus*). It is a cooling herb with a p*itta*-balancing effect. Ayurveda believes that balancing the *doshas* affects one's mood.
- *Bacopa* is another *pitta*-balancing herb that has shown

promise in the treatment of depression. Begin with 350–400 mg per day and gradually increase to 800 mg per day if it is tolerated well.
- *Ginkgo biloba* is a calming herb with neuroprotective properties. Take 120–240 mg per day. These seem to extend (at least in part) to mood. If you are taking a blood thinner, such as aspirin, or if you've been diagnosed with a bleeding condition, don't take it.
- Begin consuming cilantro (a handful per day) and coriander seeds (one teaspoon per meal) on a daily basis. Both are cooling, and cilantro is detoxifying, especially if you've been exposed to a lot of heavy metals.
- Consider a well-planned detox regimen that includes liver-supporting herbs.
- *Pitta* is balanced by sweet tastes and fragrances such as rose and other flowers. Diffusing rose essential oil or applying it to the skin with a carrier oil on a regular basis will help to stabilize *pitta*.
- *Arjuna*, an Ayurvedic herb, may help to stabilize *sadhaka pitta*, the *pitta* component that regulates emotions.

Worry, restlessness, insomnia, and a feeling of imbalance are all symptoms of *vata* depression, which is marked by an excess of the stress hormone cortisol. New mothers with *vata* depression have usually pushed themselves (or felt pushed) beyond their limits and have become exhausted as a result. This is similar to a nervous breakdown and is often compared to an anxiety-depressive condition. This state has a strong ruminative component which is characterized by an inability to turn off the mind. Grounding, warming, and soothing qualities are key for resolving *vata* depression (Budd, 2020).

- Plan for 15–30 minutes of yoga and 15–30 minutes of seated meditation per day. *Vata* benefits greatly from consistency and concentration.
- Since loneliness is a common symptom of *vata* depression, schedule at least one social activity per week.
- *Vata* is fundamentally ungrounded, so it is important to maintain a connection to nature. Spending 30 minutes or more per day outside and doing simple things like sitting on the grass, or gardening can be extremely beneficial.
- Soft, nourishing whole foods like soup, rice porridge, and baked vegetables should be consumed more frequently. Reduce cold foods and avoid dry, processed foods (like chips or crackers; salads and smoothies).
- Consume two tablespoons of loose *tulsi* (holy basil) tea three or four times a day. Take 800–1,000 mg per day in capsule form as an alternative.
- Passionflower is included in the *vata* segment because it is soothing to the nervous system. It has a growing body of evidence to back up its use for anxiety.
- Chamomile is a good option for depression caused by *vata*. High doses may be a little drying, but moderate doses have a calming effect. Aim for doses of 250–500 mg per day. In proper quantities, it can also help with depression.
- The Ayurvedic herb *jatamansi* has been used as a *vata* balancer for centuries, with doses varying from 450 to 1,000

mg per day. It is widely used to treat anxiety and insomnia. It may also have moderate anti-depressant properties.
- While *Ashwagandha* was mentioned in the *kapha* portion, it is also a good *vata* balancer. As a result, it deserves to be included in the Ayurvedic treatment of *vata* or *kapha* depression at doses of 350–800 mg per day.
- *Gotu Kola* is beneficial to all *doshas*, but it is included here especially because it has the best evidence for use with anxiety. There have been no human studies on *gotu kola* for depression, but there have been several rodent studies that indicate it may help; consider a dosage of 700–1,400 mg/day.
- Daily probiotics are beneficial for all *doshas*, but particularly for *vata* and *kapha*, which have weaker digestion than *pitta*.
- Turmeric has gained a lot of attention as a result of its substantial clinically reported effectiveness in treating depression at doses of 1,500–2,000 mg/day. Add black pepper to taste. Long-term high doses can aggravate *vata* and *pitta*, but short-term use is beneficial to all *doshas*.
- Self-massage with a warming oil can be done on a regular basis (sesame or almond).
- Encourage restful sleep by putting your child to bed around 10 p.m. If necessary, use herbs to help with this. *Ashwagandha*, passionflower, *tulsi*, and *jatamansi* are among the herbs that can support this (Budd, 2020).

Postpartum Hemorrhage

You may also be having trouble with postpartum hemorrhage. If this is happening, there are some herbal remedies that you can consider.

Remember to only consume this after professional advice and approval, and only go for the organic variants to avoid pesticide consumption (James-Parham, 2014):

- Anti-septic, anti-spasmodic, anti-bacterial, styptic, and tonic, Capsicum/cayenne pepper is used for pain relief, as a stimulant, and for postpartum hemorrhage prevention.
- Astringent, stimulant, and emetic, Bayberry/Wax Myrtle Root Bark (*Myrica cerifera*) is used to treat uterine hemorrhage.
- Astringent Yarrow (*Achillea millefolium*) is used to treat slow-healing wounds and avoid excessive bleeding.
- Blue Cohosh/Squawroot Root (*Caulophyllum thalictroides*) is anti-spasmodic and a uterine tonic. It is used to stimulate uterine contractions, relieve labor pains, and treat amenorrhea and dysmenorrhea.
- Astringent, depurative, styptic, and an emmenagogue, Lady's Mantle Leaf/Flower (*Alchemilla vulgaris*) is used to treat dysmenorrhea, menorrhagia, and avoid bleeding.
- Astringent, Witch Hazel Leaf/Bark (*Hamamelis virginiana*) is used for menorrhagia, aftercare in miscarriages and abortions, and to slow both internal and external bleeding.
- Motherwort Leaf/Flower (*Leonurus cardiaca*) is a sedative cardiac tonic. It is diuretic, and anti-spasmodic; it can be used to relax nerves, help with slow menstruation, and assist in placenta release.
- Angelica root (*Angelica archangelica*) is anti-spasmodic,

anti-viral, and a stimulant. It is used to induce labor and assist in the release of a retained placenta.
- Styptic and astringent, Shepherd's Purse (*Capsella bursa-pastoris*) is used to treat chronic menorrhagia and hemorrhages of all sorts.

To make a tincture to prevent hemorrhaging, combine one part Capsicum with two parts Bayberry, two parts Blue Cohosh, two parts Yarrow, one part Lady's Mantle, one part Witch Hazel, and one part Motherwort. Add this to a one-quart canning jar and fill this with 100 proof vodka. Steep anywhere from six weeks up to 12 weeks. One tincture of this would equal one dropperful (about 22 drops worth) in some warm water. Keep two drops under your tongue for two or three minutes and repeat every five minutes until bleeding has stopped or you have professional medical help at hand (James-Parham, 2014).

These remedies are designed to help you heal while maintaining your intrinsic relationship with the self. Use them with professional guidance and when needed. Trust in the healing process to work on its own. With that in mind, we are almost at the close.

CONCLUSION

Dear Reader,

This conclusion is a letter of love and compassion from me to you. You are a divine creation, capable of miraculous achievement. Everything that you have made has been the consequence of your efforts, love, and hard work. While life may seem overwhelming right now, have faith that things will get better, and you will get stronger. Remember that the aim of Ayurvedic practice is to ensure that you remain healthy and happy, both during and after your pregnancy. Due to this, we emphasize on remedies that will not have any chemical implications on your body.

The idea is to let your body heal on its own, while fortifying it with natural replenishments and plenty of rest and meditative time in nature. Give yourself time to understand how you are feeling, what you need, and what you wish to do. After you have given birth, you are in a tender place. The internal home that you made for your baby is now empty, and they are out in the world. From this time, regardless of how much you love them and protect them, they also belong to the world and not just you.

This feeling is overwhelming and can naturally throw you out of balance. Allow yourself to feel as you do but also accept that you are your own person and that you must look inward to find ultimate peace. The remedies we have discussed will fortify you, but the journey must be yours.

Childbirth is a *vata*-inducing experience, but with enough time to heal, you can easily rebalance and take on your new position. For the first 42 days, the emphasis should be on relaxation and regeneration. At this time, your husband, family members, or a postpartum midwife can take care of everyday needs so you can focus on healing and helping your baby. However, many families find it difficult to set aside this period. Spending the first two weeks after delivery in a state of full rest is recommended at the very least. Bringing the *vata dosha* into order, healing and rejuvenating the reproductive tissues (*shukra dhatu*) and encouraging good lactation channels are all priorities during this healing time (*stanya vaha srota*). These ensure that your health is taken care of and that you and your baby spend adequate time in bonding.

Use deep breathing, energetic symbolism, or a quick meditation to ground yourself before and during morning breastfeeding. For the first 42 days, avoid *asana* and other types of prolonged physical activity; however, after the first two weeks, you should take gentle, quick walks with your baby (paying attention to your body's signals and stopping if bleeding or pain worsens). Applying a small amount of *brahmi* oil to the top of the head each morning, sleeping with an eye pillow and a light scarf around the top of your head and ears, and using *apana* and *prana* hand mudras are all easy ways to relax *vata* and encourage you to be present with your infant.

Following an Ayurvedic postpartum diet is the single most important measure you will take to ensure a good postpartum recovery. It is more essential than ever to eat healthy during this delicate time of postpartum transition. It has an effect not just on your recovery but also on the health and well-being of your little one. You want your milk to be plentiful, digestible, and a nutrient-dense option, right? Good digestion is important for a speedy postpartum recovery and the production of digestible breast milk. It takes work to do this, and it doesn't just happen. The body expends an enormous amount of energy during birth, and as a result, digestion becomes weakened.

Furthermore, it takes time for your displaced organs to return to their pre-pregnancy state, making your digestion even more sensitive. In fact, your digestive system will be nearly as delicate as that of your newborn. Your diet should concentrate on cleansing and restoring your body from the effort of birthing, building digestive fire, and lactation within the first 10 days after giving birth. Soupy, hot, sticky, and moist food items should be consumed in plenty. Be sure to cook your grains and soups with more water and for longer than normal. Your rice should resemble mush! During this time, use vegetables with caution. They are all astringent, which makes them difficult to process at first. Build up the digestive fire for a few days before adding vegetables.

Consume healthy food items and modify your diet depending on the *dosha* that you need to balance. Take warm oil massages after delivering your baby. Tea made with one teaspoon of both fennel and fenugreek, decocted in four cups of water, boosts milk production and can be used for the first two weeks or longer as required. *Shatavari* powder or tablets are also good for milk production and provide nourishment (Lewin, 2018).

The proper selection, layout, and preservation of the nursery where you and your baby spend quality time is a vital part of the postpartum Ayurvedic regimen. The baby's nursery should have restricted access, be clean, and be fumigated with specific drugs. Since Ayurveda believes that both the mother and the baby have low immunity and power, this helps to avoid infections. The mention of regulating wind in the nursery is also worth noting, as *vayu* (air) levels in the mother are already considered high after birth. As a result, additional *vayu* should not be permitted to enter.

Perfect wellness, according to Ayurveda, denotes a harmony between body, mind, spirit, and the larger social environment. In reality, the Ayurvedic scriptures, thought, and practice echo the twin concepts of balance and connectedness (Vaidyam, 2017).

Ayurveda, like all holistic health systems, emphasizes the inextricable links between the body, mind, and spirit. According to Ayurvedic philosophy, everybody is born with a unique constitution known as *prakriti*. The *prakriti* is a specific combination of physical and psychological characteristics that influence how each person works. It is formed at conception (Vaidyam, 2017). As you learn to return to your roots and your baby accepts the newness of their surroundings, your aim should be to relocate your *prakriti*.

Overall, you will find that pregnancy and the period after becomes much easier when you are attuned to nature. Use this book as your guide, make your notes, scribble on it, and draw help as you need. This book is meant to help you through your journey, so wreck it with your own thoughts and ideas. The whole process is one of self-realization. I am honored to have been of some help along the way, but now it is time for you to begin. This will be an amazing journey, so enjoy every minute of it. Welcome to your future!

REFERENCES

6 Different Types of Taste & Their Roles According to Ayurveda. (n.d.). Dabur: Celebrate Life. Retrieved May 7, 2021, from https://www.dabur.com/in/en-us/about/science-of-ayurveda/Ayurvedic-diet/types-of-tastes#:~:text=Astringent taste&text=Their unique property reflects in,make up the kapha dosha.

Ayurvedic Tips for A Healthy Menstrual Cycle. (2018). Vedicine. https://www.vedicine.org/2018/10/ayurveda-healthy-menstrual-cycle.html

Bagde, A., Ukhalkar, V., J., P., D., B., & Sawant, R. (2013). Ayurvedic Approach for Conceiving a Healthy Progeny. *International Research Journal of Pharmacy, 4.*

Bliss, S. (2017). *Ayurvedic Subdoshas and how best to Nourish them*. Basmati. https://basmati.com/2017/04/11/Ayurvedic-sub-doshas-and-how-best-nourish-them

Budd, K. (2020). *Ayurvedic Approach to Dealing with Depression*. Chopra. https://chopra.com/articles/Ayurvedic-approach-to-dealing-with-depression

Chowdhury, R. R. (2021). *Ayurveda 101: Seven Dhatus*. The Art of Living. https://artoflivingretreatcenter.org/blog/ayurveda-101-seven-dhatus/

Dashiell, E. (2020). *Three Types of Dosha Metabolic Types in Ayurveda*. Verywellhealth. https://www.verywellhealth.com/what-is-a-dosha-88832

Data & Statistics on Birth Defects. (2020). The National Center on Birth Defects and Developmental Disabilities. https://www.cdc.gov/ncbddd/birthdefects/data.html

Doshas & The 6 Tastes. (2018). Deacon. https://doshaguru.com/doshas-the-6-tastes/

Douillard, J. (2020). *Ayurvedic Approach to Fertility, Pregnancy +PostPartum Care*. Lifespa. https://lifespa.com/ayurveda-fertility/

Girija, P. (2013). *Jeevani- Ayurveda for Women*. Sanjeevani Ayurveda Foundation.

Goenka, S. N. (2021). *Vipassana Meditation*. Dhamma.Org. https://www.dhamma.org/en/about/vipassana

Goodreads. (n.d.). *A quote from Essential Ayurveda*. Goodreads. https://www.goodreads.com/quotes/1180769-the-great-thing-about-ayurveda-is-that-its-treatments-always.

Halpern, M. (2010). *The Five Elements: Ether in Ayurveda*. California College of Ayurveda. https://www.ayurvedacollege.com/blog/five-elements-ether-ayurveda/

Hope-Murray, A. (2021). *The Three Doshas in Ayurveda*. John Wiley & Sons. https://www.dummies.com/health/the-three-doshas-in-ayurveda/

Infertility management in Ayurveda. (2019). Vikaspedia. https://vikaspedia.in/health/ayush/ayurveda-1/infertility

Jagyasi, P. (2021). *Hot and cold foods: A guide to Ayurvedic diet*. DIY Health. https://diyhealth.com/hot-and-cold-foods-a-guide-to-Ayurvedic-diet.html

James-Parham, M. (2014). *Herbs For Postpartum Hemorrhage*. Midwitchery. https://www.midwitchery.net/post/herbs-for-postpartum-hemorrhage

Karamchedu, S. (2013). *Women's Infertility- An Ayurvedic Perspective*. https://www.ayurvedacollege.com/wp-content/uploads/2017/06/Womens-Infertility-SirishaKaramchedu.pdf

Khatri, V. (2011). *The Difference Between Ayurveda and Modern Medicine*. Illuminated Health. https://illuminatedhealth.com/the-difference-between-ayurveda-and-modern-medicine/

Lad, V. (2002). *Introduction to Panchakarma*. The Ayurvedic Institute. https://www.ayurveda.com/resources/cleansing/introduction-to-panchakarma

Lad, V. (2016). *Ayurveda: A Brief Introduction and Guide.*

Lewin, M. (2018). *Sweet Blessings: Ayurvedic Postpartum Care.* Banyan. https://www.banyanbotanicals.com/info/blog-banyan-vine/details/sweet-blessings-Ayurvedic-postpartum-care/

Mahatyagi, R. Das. (2013). *Ayurvedic Treatment for Spotting or Vaginal Bleeding Between Periods.* Yatan. https://www.yatan-ayur.com.au/spotting-vaginal-bleeding-between-periods/#:~:text=When no medical condition is,to manufacture its own hormones.

Mischke, M. (2020). *Ama: The Antithesis of Agni.* Banyan. https://www.banyanbotanicals.com/info/Ayurvedic-living/living-ayurveda/health-guides/understanding-agni/ama-the-antithesis-of-agni/

Naturally Sweet Foods: The Most Satvik Of All As Per Ayurveda. (2019). Ayiurvedam Editorial. https://www.ayurvedum.com/sweet-food/

Ojas. (2015). Maharshi Ayurveda. http://www.ayurveda.org.au/ojas/

Parker, J. (2021). *What Are The 5 Elements of Ayurveda And What They Mean.* Mother of Health. https://motherofhealth.com/the-5-elements-of-ayurveda

Pashte, S. (2017). Concept of Human Embryology, Foetal Growth and Development. *International Journal of Applied Ayurved Research, June.*

Prana in Food. (2017). Ayurvedic Way of Living. https://svasthyagyan.wordpress.com/2017/10/09/prana-in-food/

Reist, P. L. (2018). *The Basics of Ayurveda: The Earth Element.* The Art of Living. https://www.artofliving.org/in-en/basics-ayurveda-earth-element

Simplify Your Pregnancy with Ayurveda. (2020). Art of Living. https://artoflivingretreatcenter.org/blog/simplify-your-pregnancy-with-ayurveda/

Stages of labor and birth: Baby, it's time! (2020). Mayo Clinic. https://www.mayoclinic.org/healthy-lifestyle/labor-and-delivery/in-depth/stages-of-labor/art-20046545

Swati. (2021). *Top 5 Herbs For Balancing Apana Vata: Ayurvedic Apana Vata Herbs.* Honey Fur. https://honeyfurforher.com/top-Ayurvedic-herbs-for-balancing-apana-vata-vayu/

The 20 Gunas. (2020). Wasatch Ayurveda and Yoga. https://www.wasatchayurvedaandyoga.com/the-20-gunas/

The Ayurvedic Doshas. (2021). Kripalu Yoga. https://kripalu.org/resources/Ayurvedic-doshas

The six tastes of Ayurveda. (2021). Pukka. https://uk.pukkaherbs.com/wellbeing-articles/the-six-tastes-of-ayurveda#:~:text=Balancing the doshas,volume of all the tissues.

Vaidyam, S. (2017). *Ayurvedic post partum regimen: first person account by Seetha Vaidyam.* Krya. https://krya.in/2017/01/Ayurvedic-post-natal-care-to-strengthen-nourish-and-care-for-a-new-mother-and-a-new-born-baby-krya-shares-a-first-person-account/

What's my Vikruti? Classic Signs of Imbalance in each of the Doshas. (2018). Bright Body. https://mybrightbody.com/blogs/blog/whats-my-vikruti-classic-signs-of-imbalance-in-each-of-the-doshas#:~:text=Classic Signs of Imbalance in each of the Doshas,-February 23%2C 2018&text=Typically%2C the dosha that is,to bring back into balance.

Wolf, J. (2016). *What is the best oil for your Dosha?* The Lotus Room. https://www.thelotusroomnashville.com/living-ayurveda/2016/10/5/what-is-the-best-oil-for-your-dosha

Wong, C. (2020). *Three Types of Dosha Metabolic Types in Ayurveda.* Verywellhealth. https://www.verywellhealth.com/what-is-a-dosha-88832

Made in the USA
Las Vegas, NV
21 March 2025